HUMAN ORAL MUCOSA

HUMAN ORAL MUCOSA

DEVELOPMENT, STRUCTURE AND FUNCTION

CHRISTOPHER A. SQUIER
NEWELL W. JOHNSON
ROSAMUND M. HOPPS

Department of Oral Pathology
The London Hospital Medical College
London E.1

BLACKWELL SCIENTIFIC PUBLICATIONS
OXFORD LONDON EDINBURGH MELBOURNE

© 1976 Blackwell Scientific Publications
Osney Mead, Oxford,
8 John Street, London, WC1
9 Forrest Road, Edinburgh,
P.O. Box 9, North Balwyn, Victoria, Australia.

First published 1976

British Library Cataloguing in Publication Data
Squier, Christopher A.
    Human oral mucosa: development, structure and function.
    Bibl.—Index.
    ISBN 0-632-00751-6
    1. Title 2. Johnson, Newell W.
    3. Hopps, Rosamund M.
    612'.31   QP146
    Mouth
    Mucous membrane

Distributed in the United States of America by
J.B. Lippincott Company, Philadelphia,
and in Canada by
J.B. Lippincott Company of Canada Ltd., Toronto.

Phototypeset by Oliver Burridge Filmsetting Limited, Crawley
Printed in Great Britain by
the Alden Press, Oxford
and bound by
Kemp Hall Bindery

CONTENTS

ACKNOWLEDGEMENTS

We are grateful to those people who have willingly given advice in the writing of this book or who have read the manuscript and offered constructive criticisms; in particular we thank Julia Meyer, Susan Tinkler, and John Clement. John Linder has contributed greatly by the preparation both of original histological material and in the production of micrographs. Finally we would like to express our appreciation to Mrs V. Mulligan who so cheerfully typed the manuscript.

INTRODUCTION

The oral mucosa is all too frequently regarded by the
dentist as no more than the soft tissues surrounding his
principal target, the teeth, for it is the teeth themselves
and their supporting tissues that show the most common
oral diseases–dental caries and periodontal disease. On
the other hand, the dermatologist sees many skin lesions
that also involve areas of the oral mucous membrane and
so considers it essentially as an extension of the skin into
the oral cavity. The physician appreciates the diagnostic
value of the oral mucosa in recognizing many forms of
systemic disease, including those involving the gut
mucosa, and also uses it at times as an efficient means of
systemic drug delivery. All these attitudes reflect important properties of the oral mucosa yet it is rare to find
a unified account of this organ in which these different
attributes are considered.

In many ways the mucosa lining the oral cavity is
intermediate between the skin covering the outside of the
body and the mucous membrane lining of the rest of the
alimentary canal. Like the skin the oral mucosa has an
epithelium comprising several layers of closely packed
cells, the surface of which forms a horny barrier in some
regions. Supporting this is a connective tissue containing
ground substance, fibres and cells, the properties of
which reflect the functional demands of the region.
There is a sensory innervation that makes some areas,
such as the tip of the tongue, at least as sensitive to

1

tactile stimuli as the fingertips, yet the oral mucosa is able to withstand temperatures that feel uncomfortably warm to the skin.

On the other hand, appendages such as hair follicles and sweat glands that are abundant in skin are absent from oral mucosa, although there are numerous salivary glands that are responsible for maintaining its characteristically moist surface. In this latter respect it resembles the rest of the intestinal tract, as does its rapid rate of cell renewal and the presence of areas that lack a horny surface.

In this volume we have tried to provide a more comprehensive account of the oral mucosa than is found in most of the standard texts on histology and dental anatomy by pointing out its similarities and differences to both skin and other mucous membranes and by emphasizing how it fulfils the various functional demands made on it às the lining of the oral cavity. We first describe the functions of the oral mucosa and then go on to explain how the structure fulfils the functions. While the first chapters provide an overview of the complete organ, the later chapters go into more detail and include descriptions of fine structure, biochemistry and physiology—these should be intelligible to students who are taking courses in the basic sciences relevant to dentistry or medicine. Finally there is an account of how epithelium and mesenchymal tissues interact, and of the development and ageing of the oral mucosa. Much of the information in this book is necessarily based on the findings of many research workers in oral biology; for the sake of continuity we have not cited references to support each statement of fact but have included certain key references after each chapter. At the end of the book are listed a number of publications that cover many of the topics dealt with in this volume.

CHAPTER 1
THE FUNCTIONS OF ORAL MUCOSA

Whilst the oral mucosa has some of the attributes of skin and some of intestinal mucosa, in its major functional roles of forming a protective covering layer and of conveying sensory information from the surface, it most closely resembles skin. These functions are now considered in more detail.

1:1 Protective functions

The protective role of the oral mucosa may be considered not only in terms of resistance to mechanical insult but also as restricting the entry of micro-organisms and toxic substances.

During mastication some regions of the mucosa are exposed to compression and shear forces, other regions to stretching. Both the epithelium and connective tissue show adaptations to meet these demands and as a consequence the mucosa has a different composition in different regions. For example the mucosa of the hard palate and attached gingiva has a horny surface to resist abrasion and is tightly bound to the underlying bone so as to resist shear forces; the mucosa of the cheek has a flexible surface and contains elastic tissue which allows for distension.

Large numbers of micro-organisms as well as their toxic products and other potentially harmful substances are present in the oral cavity. Their entry into the body is limited principally by the oral epithelium which forms an effective barrier layer. While there is no need, as in the skin, to restrict the loss of salts and water from the mucosal surface, as they would be recycled anyway by swallowing, there does seem to be some resistance to their outward movement. Hence the oral mucosa is not, as is sometimes suggested, a highly permeable lining membrane, but has similar barrier properties to those of epidermis although there does seem to be a weak link at the dento-gingival junction where the continuity of the epithelium is interrupted by the tooth.

1:2 Sensory functions

The oral mucosa has an important sensory function responding not only to pain, touch and temperature, as does the skin, but also to taste, a modality to which no other region of the body responds. In some ways the sensory function may be considered protective because receptors in the oral mucosa initiate swallowing, gagging and retching and the withdrawal and salivation reflexes. Finally there are receptors concerned with the so-called water taste that controls the thirst mechanism.

1:3 Other functions: thermal regulation, synthesis and secretion

The skin plays a major role in thermal regulation in which hairs, sweat glands and the local vasculature all participate. In the oral mucosa there are no hairs or sweat glands and the extent to which the blood vessels function in temperature regulation is unclear. Certainly there is heat loss from the oral mucosa of some animals under certain conditions, such as the tongue of a panting dog, and it has been suggested that a similar loss takes place from the extensive vascular anastomoses of the human sublingual region. However this is probably incidental and quantitatively insignificant.

The skin also has synthetic functions, manufacturing vitamin D, cholesterol and sebum, which is secreted. This apparently does not occur in the oral mucosa to any extent. The major secretion associated with the oral mucosa is that of the salivary glands which maintains the moist surface of the mucous membrane and assists in mastication and the passage of food and provides for some digestion of food within the oral cavity. The secretory immunoglobin system in saliva forms part of the body's defences.

Unlike the intestines, the oral mucosa has no specialized absorptive function, and though used as a route for drug administration it is probably closer to the skin than to the gut in its permeability characteristics.

CHAPTER 2
THE ORGANIZATION OF ORAL MUCOSA

The oral cavity is divided into two regions: the outer oral vestibule is bounded on the exterior by the lips and cheeks and on the interior by the maxillary and mandibular arches. The oral cavity proper is situated within the dental arches, its superior border formed by the hard and soft palates while the tongue and the floor of the mouth form the inferior border; posteriorly, the border is delineated by the pillars of the fauces and tonsils. It is sometimes difficult to envisage the location and extent of the mucosae lining these different regions and a convenient way of representing them is by means of the 'opened out' oral cavity illustrated in Fig. 1.

2:1 Clinical features of oral mucosa

Although both skin and oral mucosa have a similar histological organization there are obvious differences in their clinical appearance. The oral mucosa is moist, relatively smooth and a brighter pink than the skin; this is particularly apparent at the vermilion border of the lips where skin meets oral mucosa. The colour of the mucosa is the result of a number of interacting features; the thickness of the epithelium and its degree of keratinization and pigmentation and the concentration and state of the blood vessels in the connective tissue. Colour is often a guide to the condition of the tissue; for example inflamed gingiva appears bright red, while healthy

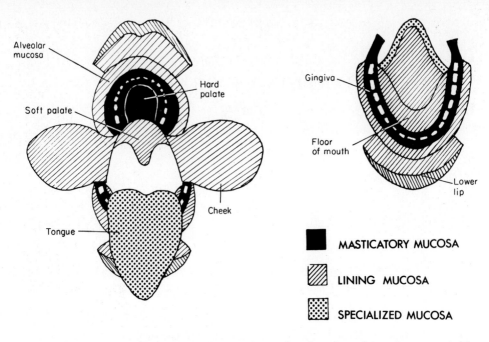

Alveolar mucosa

Hard palate

Soft palate

Tongue

Cheek

Gingiva

Floor of mouth

Lower lip

███ MASTICATORY MUCOSA

▨ LINING MUCOSA

░░ SPECIALIZED MUCOSA

Fig. 1. The oral cavity 'opened out' to show the regions occupied by masticatory, lining and specialized mucosae. (Modified from Roed-Petersen, B. & Renstrup, G. (1969). *Acta Odont Scand.* **27** 681–695.)

gingiva is a much paler pink. See Fig. 2.

The appendages found in skin are absent from oral mucosa except for the sebaceous glands, which may often be seen in the upper lip and buccal mucosa as pale yellow spots in 60–75% of adults, although they have also been reported in alveolar mucosa and the dorsum of tongue. They are sometimes referred to as Fordyce's spots or Fordyce's 'disease', though use of the term disease is unfortunate. The openings of minor salivary glands are also evident in many areas. While there are not usually many creases or wrinkles in the oral mucosa, there are characteristic surface features in several regions. The healthy gingiva shows a pattern of fine stippling (Fig. 2) representing small indentations of the epithelium while the ridges or rugae of the hard palate and the various papillae of the dorsum of the tongue (see Fig. 27) are more conspicuous topographical features.

The deformability of the mucosa, reflecting the functional demands, varies in different regions. In the gingiva and hard palate the mucosa is firm and immobile, while that of the cheek and lips is more pliable. These differences have an important bearing on surgical procedures,

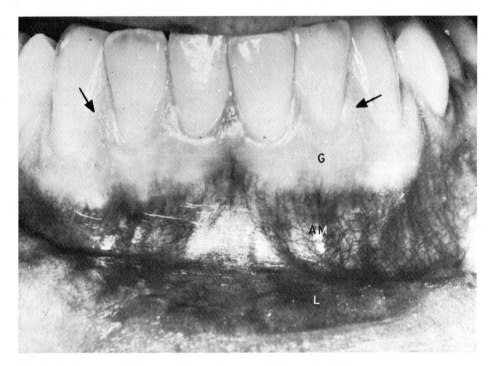

Fig. 2. A photograph showing the oral mucosa lining part of the vestibule. The gingiva (G) appears pale and stippling is visible in the interdental region (arrows). There is an abrupt junction between the gingiva and alveolar mucosa (AM) (see Fig. 29), which merges with the labial mucosa (L). Many small blood vessels can be seen in the alveolar mucosa.

incisions in the gingiva and palate requiring less suturing than in the cheek or lips which gape readily.

2:2 The component tissues and glands of oral mucosa

The oral mucosa can be most simply divided into an outer component, the *oral epithelium* which corresponds to the epidermis of skin, and an underlying connective tissue layer, the *lamina propria* or *corium* (called the dermis in skin) (Fig. 3). As in many other organs, the connective tissue plays a role both as a supporting stroma for the epithelium and as a significant tissue component with its own important functions. The junction between the epithelium and the connective tissue is represented by the *basement membrane*, a layer about 1–2 μm in thickness which although apparently structureless at the light microscope level, is a complex attachment region. This frequently appears as an undulating

9

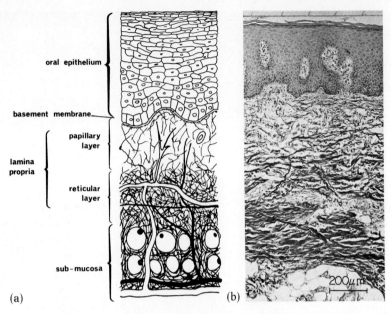

oral epithelium

basement membrane

papillary layer

lamina propria

reticular layer

sub-mucosa

200μm

(a)

(b)

Fig. 3. (a) is a diagram of the main tissue components of the oral mucosa which can all be identified in the light micrograph (b) of a histological section through the palatal mucosa.

boundary as a result of the downgrowing *epithelial ridges* or *pegs* (sometimes called 'rete ridges' or 'rete pegs') interdigitating with the *connective tissue papillae* (see Fig. 7b). Each of these major layers will be considered in more detail in succeeding chapters.

The mucous membrane lining the rest of the gastro-intestinal tract contains, in addition to the epithelium and connective tissue a third layer, the muscularis mucosae (Fig. 4a). This consists of smooth muscle and elastic tissue which separates the mucous membrane proper from the underlying connective tissue, called the *sub-mucosa*, and allows the mucosa some independence from the outer muscular wall of the gut. In the oral cavity such a layer is absent except perhaps for the soft palate and so no true sub-mucosa is recognized. However in many regions, such as the cheek, lips and parts of the hard palate, a loose fatty or glandular connective tissue containing the major blood vessels and nerves that supply the mucosa is present between the mucosa proper and underlying muscle or bone (Fig. 4b). This is some-times referred to as a sub-mucosa although it clearly does not have the same structural or functional role as that of the gut. Nevertheless because this layer is clearly 'sub-mucosal' in location, we will for convenience refer to it

10

as a sub-mucosa in this volume. In regions such as the gingiva and parts of the hard palate there is no sub-mucosal tissue and the oral mucosa is directly attached to the periostium of underlying bone; this is therefore referred to as a *muco-periostium* (Fig. 4c).

The major glandular elements associated with the oral mucosa are the salivary glands. They may be classified in various ways, according to their function, their position or their size. Most commonly they are divided on the basis of size into major and minor glands.

The major salivary glands, the parotid, the sub-mandibular (sometimes also called the submaxillary gland) and the sublingual are all large glands situated some way from the oral cavity but opening into it by long ducts. The parotid is a serous gland producing a largely watery secretion while both the submandibular and sublingual glands are mixed, the secretions being predominantly serous and mucous, respectively. Minor salivary glands are situated in or immediately beneath the oral mucosa (see Fig. 26) and are grouped together in several regions of the oral cavity. The labial glands are groups of minor glands in the upper and lower lips (see Fig. 28) and extend posteriorly into the cheek to form the buccal glands; both groups of glands are predominantly mucous secreting. The glossopalatine glands, situated in

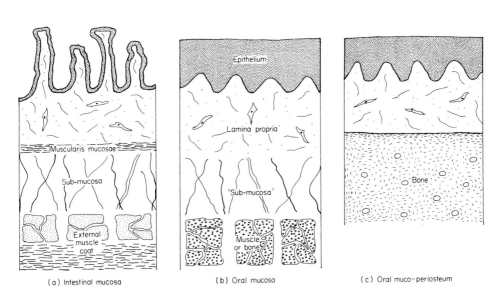

(a) Intestinal mucosa   (b) Oral mucosa   (c) Oral muco-periosteum

Fig. 4. Diagram to show the arrangement of the different tissue components in (a) intestinal mucosa, (b) oral mucosa and (c) oral muco-periosteum.

11

the glossopalatine folds and oro-pharyngeal isthmus of the tongue, and the palatine glands of the hard palate, soft palate and uvula are pure mucous glands, as are the lingual glands on the ventral surface of the anterior part of the tongue. The posterior lingual glands at the base of the tongue are mucous secreting, while those around the vallate papillae, von Ebners glands, are serous.

The sebaceous glands, when present, lie in the lamina propria of the mucosa and are similar in structure to those associated with hair follicles in skin where they produce sebum, a fatty secretion that probably emulsifies with sweat and forms a film coating the skin surface. Their function in oral mucosa is unknown and they may merely represent areas of ectoderm retaining some of the potential of skin from embryological development.

In the posterior region of the oral cavity are large accumulations of lymphoid tissue forming the lingual, palatine and pharyngeal tonsils; they are collectively referred to as Waldeyers ring. The tonsils represent deep crypts in the lamina propria into which the overlying epithelium is invaginated and extensively infiltrated with lymphocytes, plasma cells and neutrophilic leucocytes. Small lymphoid nodules may also occur in the mucosa of the soft palate, the ventral surface of tongue and the floor of mouth. This tissue by virtue of its ability to mount immunological reactions plays an important role in combating infection.

2:3 The cell types of oral mucosa

The structure and organization of mammalian cells are frequently described in terms of a generalized cell such as that shown in Fig. 5a, which contains a representative collection of the organelles that are encountered in the cells of most tissues. While this is a convenient way of illustrating cell ultrastructure it is an oversimplification, and before discussing the cell types making up the oral mucosa it is worth pointing out a distinction between two major sorts of cell—those primarily concerned with the synthesis of material for secretion ('secretors') and those that retain most of their synthetic products ('retainers'). In the former type, the organelles most concerned with the synthesis, packaging and export of cell products predominate (Fig. 5b). There is abundant rough

12

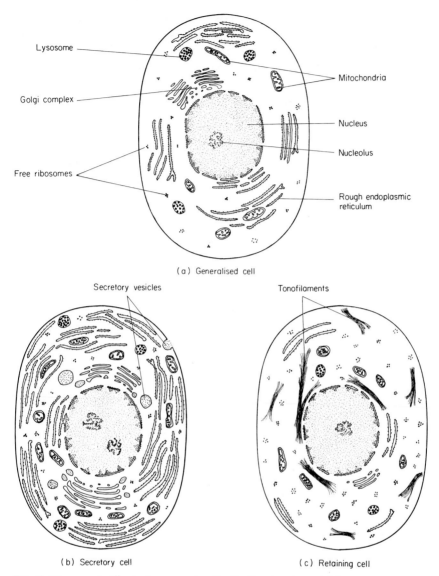

Lysosome

Golgi complex

Free ribosomes

Mitochondria

Nucleus

Nucleolus

Rough endoplasmic reticulum

(a) Generalised cell

Secretory vesicles

Tonofilaments

(b) Secretory cell

(c) Retaining cell

Fig. 5. Diagram to illustrate concepts of cell ultrastructure. (a) is a generalized cell while the secretory cell (b) and the retaining cell (c) represent extremes of functional specialization (see text).

endoplasmic reticulum, a well developed Golgi system and numerous secretory vesicles; mitochondria are plentiful. Typical examples of the secretory cell type are those cells present in the pancreatic and salivary acini. Retaining cells, on the other hand, have far less rough endoplasmic reticulum and smaller Golgi systems (Fig. 5c). Here synthesis is mainly directed to producing structural elements that will be retained by the cell, and this can take place on free ribosomes, so 'packaging' by a

13

Golgi system is unnecessary. Lower energy requirements mean that mitochondria are small and infrequent. The retained synthetic product may be visible within the cell; in the extreme example of the erythrocyte this is haemoglobin, which entirely fills the mature cell, while in fully differentiated keratinized cells such as those of the surface layer of the epidermis, it is keratin.

The oral mucosa displays two extremes of cellular organization. The epithelium is highly cellular, consisting of tightly apposed retaining cells separated by a minimum of intercellular substance, whose principal synthetic activity (apart from the production of intercellular material) is to manufacture the characteristic fibrillar protein retained within the cell. Since this protein forms the basic material from which a keratin layer may arise, such epithelial cells are often referred to as *keratinocytes*. In addition there are occasional cells with other specific functions, such as the secretion of pigment. The structure and function of these epithelial cell types are described more fully in the next chapter. The connective tissue of the lamina propria, on the other hand, is relatively acellular and consists principally of a ground substance in which are situated fibrous protein elements—predominantly collagen, and the cells responsible for secreting both ground substance and fibres—the fibroblasts (or fibrocytes) which are typical secretor type cells. The ground substance, like the intercellular substance of the epithelium, consists of 'mucosubstances' i.e. macro-molecular protein-carbohydrate complexes, whose composition varies depending on the region from which the tissue comes and on its metabolic and physiological state. The structure and classification of these substances is described in Appendix 2. Intimately associated with the outer aspect of the membrane of all cell types is a unique layer of mucosubstance—the cell coat or glycocalyx. This seems to confer a specificity on the cell which is recognized by the cellular and humoral components of the immune system. As well as fibroblasts there are of course a variety of cells concerned with maintenance and defence of the connective tissue, such as mast cells, tissue macrophages and wandering leucocytes. Most of these cells fall between the extreme types of secretor and retainer represented by the keratinocyte and the fibroblast, and will be described more fully in Chapter 4.

14

Further reading

MASON D.K. & CHISHOLM D.M. (1975) *Salivary glands in health and disease.* W.B. Saunders Co. Ltd., London.

MERCER E.H. (1964) Protein synthesis and epidermal differentiation. In *The Epidermis* (edited by Montagna, W. and Lobitz, W.C.) Academic Press, New York.

MILES A.E.W. (1963) Sebaceous glands in oral and lip mucosa. In *Advances in Biology of Skin* (edited by Montagna, W., Ellis, R.A. and Silver, A.F.) 1–32, Pergamon Press, Oxford.

CHAPTER 3
THE EPITHELIUM

The epithelial lining of the oral mucosa forms a protective covering for the tissues beneath and a barrier to the entry of foreign material and micro-organisms. These functions are reflected by the organization of the epithelium in which individual epithelial cells are closely apposed and stratified so there are a number of layers which show a sequence of differentiation, the most superficial layers forming a surface resistant to physical insult and to penetration by foreign substances. There is a constant loss of cells from the surface as a result of wear and tear, and as the differentiating cells are incapable of division, it is the relatively undifferentiated cells in or near the basal layer that provide replacements. This chapter describes the processes of division and differentiation that contribute to epithelial homeostasis and also deals with the non-epithelial cell types invariably found in the epithelium.

3:1 Cell division and tissue turnover

The epithelium lining the oral mucosa, like that of the rest of the gastro-intestinal tract and the epidermis, is composed of a constantly renewing cell population in which, under normal circumstances, the number of new cells produced by division in the basal region is just sufficient to match those lost by desquamation at the surface.

17

There has been some disagreement over the exact site of cell division in oral epithelium and consequently as to what constitutes the *germinative layers* or *progenitor cell compartment*. However this was resolved by examining serial sections of epithelium when almost all dividing cells were found to lie on the basement membrane or within three cell layers of it. It was also thought for many years that the distribution of dividing cells along the basement membrane was random, but it is now clear that they frequently occur in regular clusters, and in epithelium with a complex connective tissue interface (such as the attached gingiva) cell divisions are more numerous at the tips of the rete pegs.

It is customary to divide the life span of dividing cells into a number of phases (Fig. 6). The histologically distinct stages of mitosis (prophase, metaphase, anaphase and telophase) are collectively known as the M phase. Mitotic division is followed by a post-mitotic resting period or gap, G1. The extra DNA required for division is synthesized during S phase. This is separated from the period of mitosis proper by a premitotic gap, G2. G1, together with S and G2, are histologically undetectable events occurring during interphase. Between M and G1 is the so-called dichophase, a period of indeterminate length during which each daughter cell 'makes the decision' to remain part of the progenitor population or to begin differentiation and so eventually reach the surface layers. Estimates for the time taken for an epithelial cell to pass through S, G2 and M vary from 9 to 11 hours,

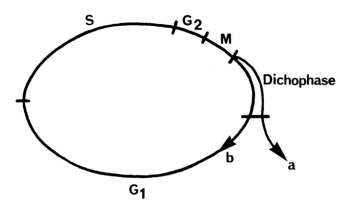

Fig. 6. Phases of the cell cycle.
(a) daughter cell proceeding to differentiation.
(b) daughter cell remaining as part of progenitor population (see text for other symbols).

18

mitotic division itself taking 30–60 min, while the duration of the resting period gap G1 is more variable, being between 14 and 140 hours.

Although it is sometimes useful to know the total time taken for a cell to pass through the entire mitotic cycle, a more valuable parameter is the proportion of cells in the epithelium which are dividing at any given time – the *mitotic index*. This can be determined readily if 'stathmokinetic' chemicals such as the plant alkaloid colchicine are administered to block mitoses at metaphase. The numbers of mitotic figures accumulating in a given period enable the mitotic index to be calculated. Alternatively, if radioactively labelled DNA precursors, such as tritiated thymidine, are administered to the tissue then the nuclei of cells in S phase will appear labelled in subsequent autoradiographs. This provides a *labelling index* which is an estimate of the number of cells preparing for division. Obviously indices of this sort can be expressed in various ways and the number of dividing or labelled cells has been related to various baselines such as the total number of nucleated epithelial cells in a given area, or to the number of basal cells in a given area, or alternatively to unit length of basement membrane or unit area of desquamating epithelial surface. This latter index is probably most useful in describing the behaviour of the tissue as, under steady state conditions, cell division must be just sufficient to replace cells shed at the epithelial surface. However in practice the overriding requirement is that the type of index used should be clearly understood.

One of the problems in dealing with a stratified epithelium is that a mitotic index does not describe fully events taking place in the whole tissue. For example, even though the number of dividing cells increases, the number undergoing differentiation and migrating to the surface may not increase, so that the epithelial population may well just show a change in the ratio of progenitor to differentiating cells and thus become thicker. Alternatively, the rate of differentiation, migration, and of cell desquamation may accelerate without any change in mitotic index, so that the epithelium in fact becomes thinner. Such changes can be identified by measuring epithelial thickness or by counting the number of cell layers.

An alternative way of expressing the dynamic events in a renewing cell population is to calculate *turnover*

Table 1. Total tissue turnover times for different regions of human oral epithelia, compared to that of skin. Data derived from that quoted in Oral Mucosa in Health and Disease (edited by Dolby, A.E.) Chapter 1. Blackwell Scientific Publications, Oxford, 1975.

	DAYS	
	Median	Range
Skin	27	12–75
Buccal Mucosa (non-keratinized	14	5–16
Hard Palate (keratinized)	24	–
Floor of Mouth (non-keratinized)	20	–
Gingiva—oral aspect of free and attached gingiva (keratinized)	11*	8–40
Oral sulcular epithelium	6*	4–10

*Indicates data from non-human primate.

time, which may be defined as the time taken for the total number of cells in the tissue to be shed and replaced by an equal number of cells through division. Measurement of turnover time will thus require a knowledge of the time a cell spends in the mitotic cycle as well as of the time taken for a cell to migrate through the entire thickness of the epithelium (transit time). It is then assumed that under steady state conditions one of the two daughter cells arising from each division remains part of the progenitor compartment and the other begins the process of differentiation and migration towards the surface. These assumptions are not always justified and so the turnover time, like the mitotic index, can only be an approximate expression of tissue behaviour. Despite the many difficulties in obtaining measurements of the cellular dynamics of stratified epithelia, there is some general agreement as to turnover times for a variety of different tissues. In general oral epithelium turns over faster than epidermis but more slowly than gut epithelium; estimates for this vary between 4 and 14 days. Between different regions of the oral mucosa there are also variations in epithelial turnover times; these are set out in Table 1, from which it is clear that the non-keratinized lining mucosa of the cheek turns over faster than the keratinized masticatory mucosa of the attached gingiva and hard palate.

The control of cell division is thought to be brought about by locally produced tissue hormones termed *chalones*. These, it is suggested, are produced by post-mitotic epithelial cells and have the dual property of stimulating cell differentiation and inhibiting mitosis— cell division is thus highest in regions of low chalone concentration. A systemic component is also involved in chalone action and this is claimed to be adrenalin. A number of other factors influence mitotic activity, the most important of which are the effect of diurnal rhythm, stress and age. Endocrine status and the presence of inflammation variously affect epithelial mitotic rates; for example in the gingiva, which is invariably inflamed, a small inflammatory infiltrate stimulates mitosis while larger infiltrates appear to depress mitotic activity.

3:2 Stratification and the characteristic layers of the epithelium

Cells arising by division in the basal region of the epithelium undergo a process of differentiation to form a protective surface layer. This process is not identical in the various regions of the oral mucosa, and as a consequence we can recognize different types of surface that reflect different patterns of differentiation. The surface layers may generally be divided into three types described as ortho-keratinized (Fig. 7a), para-keratinized (Fig. 7b) and non-keratinized (Fig. 7c). However, whatever the surface appearance, we can recognize similar patterns of differentiation in the deep part of the epithelium in all regions. The deepest epithelial cells are cuboidal or columnar cells, in contact with the basement membrane and forming the *basal layer* or *stratum basale*. These cells are primarily responsible for division and replacement of cells lost at the surface and while it is possible to classify them functionally as a germinative layer (or stratum germinativum) this is not altogether desirable because, as we have already mentioned, some cell division does take place supra-basally. Above the basal layer are several layers of larger cells, which may be isodiametric or slightly flattened and which, because of the 'spiky' appearance of their intercellular attachments in histological preparations (see Fig. 16) are called prickle cells. These constitute the *prickle cell layer* or *stratum spinosum*.

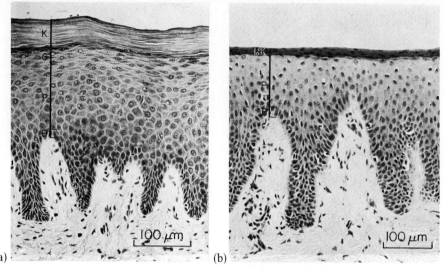

(a)   (b)

Fig. 7. Types of surface epithelium seen in human oral mucosa.

(a) ortho-keratinized epithelium from the hard palate; a prominent granular layer is present.

(b) para-keratinized epithelium from the gingiva; a granular layer is not readily apparent and pyknotic nuclei are present in the surface layer. Note the well defined epithelial pegs.

(c) non-keratinized epithelium from buccal mucosa; the epithelium is considerably thicker than that in (a) or (b) and nuclei are present up to the surface layers. (B = basal layer; P = prickle cell layer; G = granular layer; K = keratinized layer; PK = para-keratinized layer; I = intermediate layer; S = superficial layer).

The basal and prickle cell layers together constitute approximately half to two-thirds of the thickness of the epithelium, and it is only in the remaining layers that clear differences in the pathways of differentiation emerge (Fig. 7).

In regions of the oral mucosa that are designated as keratinized, the prickle cell layer is succeeded by larger but more flattened cells which contain numbers of basophilic keratohyalin granules, and constitute the *granular layer* or *stratum granulosum*. All the cell layers so far mentioned contain nucleated cells and the term *Malpighian layer* is sometimes used to describe these strata collectively. The most superficial layer is the *ortho-keratinized, cornified* or *horny layer*. The cells are markedly flattened consisting of hexagonal discs, termed squames, filled with eosinophilic material representing the keratin. Although a 'stratum lucidum' is recognized between the granular and keratinized layers of the epidermis this is not often seen in oral epithelium. In *para-keratinized*

22

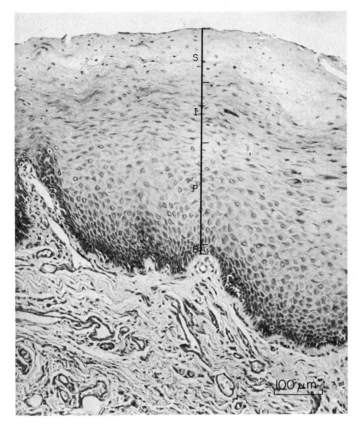

Fig. 7(c)

epithelium the surface cells, while staining for keratin
with eosin and other acidophilic dyes, retain shrunken
(pyknotic) nuclei, and a distinct granular layer is often
difficult to recognize or is absent.

It is more difficult to divide the outer layers of *non-
keratinized* oral epithelium into clear cut histological zones
because this tissue lacks a granular layer and the surface
cells retain apparently normal nuclei and show little or
no eosinophilia. However, the outer third to one half of
the epithelium may be divided equally but rather arbi-
trarily into the *intermediate* and the *superficial layers*. As
we will mention in the next section there is some justifi-
cation at the ultrastructural level for distinguishing these
two layers.

Apart from differences in their surface layers, keratinized and non-keratinized epithelia also differ in their
epithelial ridge pattern, that of non-keratinized epithelia
being relatively short and blunt. Non-keratinized epithelia are also thicker, often being as much as twice the

23

thickness of keratinized epithelia. These differences are described in more detail in Chapter 6.

3:3 Patterns of differentiation in oral epithelium

It has already been pointed out that the major function of the oral epithelium is to form a protective surface layer, and that this surface has different characteristics in different regions. To produce a surface with the appropriate properties the epithelial cell undergoes a process of differentiation as it moves upwards from the basal layer. This is a well ordered process and successive epithelial layers contain cells of increasing age which are at advancing stages of maturation (Fig. 8).

The basal epithelial cells (Fig. 9) represent the least differentiated cells of the epithelium; they possess not only the usual organelles seen in other cell types but also some characteristic features such as *tonofilaments* that distinguish them from the cells of most other tissues. The tonofilaments are fine intracellular protein strands, some 8 nm in diameter which, when arranged together in bundles, form *tonofibrils* visible with the higher powers of the light microscope. These filaments represent a synthetic product, retained within the cell as a structural element, as described in Chapter 2, section 3.

The effectiveness of the epithelium as a barrier depends greatly on cohesion between individual epithelial cells and on the adhesion of the whole epithelium to underlying tissues. Cohesion is promoted by the presence of an intercellular mucosubstance composed of protein-polysaccharide complexes of the sort generally classified as proteoglycans (see Appendix 2) which are one of the few secretory products of the epithelial cells. More important in providing cell to cell attachment are the characteristic structural modifications of the plasma membranes which form the intercellular junctions (Fig. 10).

The *desmosome* is the most common of these, occupying oval or circular areas of adjacent plasma membranes, where intracellular thickening can be seen forming attachment plaques into which the cytoplasmic tonofilaments are inserted. In the intercellular region between these plaques are light and dark lamellae. During histological processing the epithelial cells tend to shrink except where they are held together by the desmosomes,

24

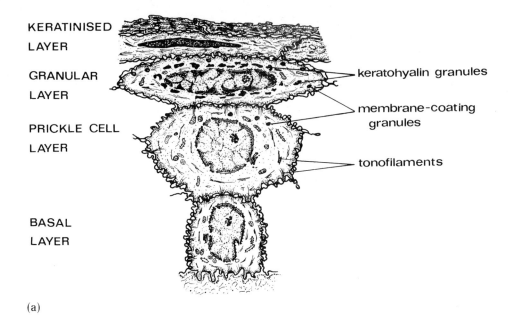

KERATINISED LAYER

GRANULAR LAYER — keratohyalin granules

— membrane-coating granules

PRICKLE CELL LAYER — tonofilaments

BASAL LAYER

(a)

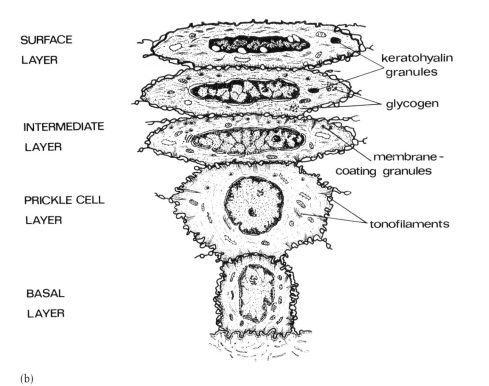

SURFACE LAYER — keratohyalin granules

— glycogen

INTERMEDIATE LAYER

— membrane-coating granules

PRICKLE CELL LAYER — tonofilaments

BASAL LAYER

(b)

Fig. 8. Diagrams to show the main characteristics of successive cell layers in (a) ortho-keratinized and (b) non-keratinized oral epithelium (see text for details).

25

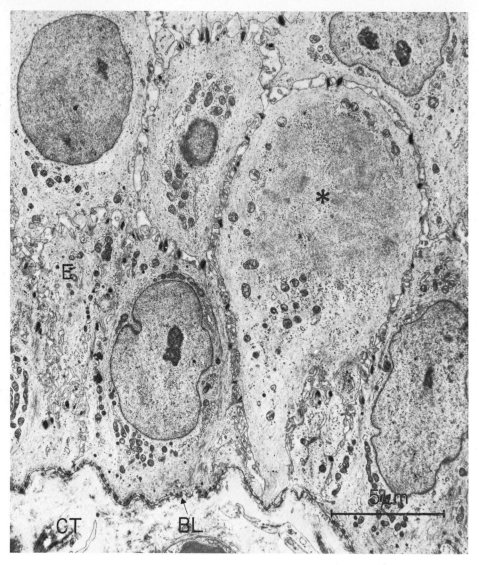

Fig. 9. Electron micrograph of basal cells from buccal epithelium. One of the basal cells (asterisk) is beginning to divide and has lost its nuclear membrane. Tonofilaments are sparse but mitochondria are visible in all cells. The basement lamina (BL) separating the epithelium (E) from the connective tissue (CT) is clearly seen.

so producing the appearance of intercellular bridges in the 'prickle cell' layer, although it is clear that no cytoplasmic continuity exists between adjacent epithelial cells. Adhesion between the epithelium and the underlying connective tissue is mediated by *hemi-desmosomes* arranged along the basal plasma membrane of the basal cells (see Fig. 25); these also possess intracellular attachment plaques into which tonofilaments are inserted. The structure of this zone is described more fully in Chapter 5. Desmosomes represent a mechanical link between cells so that localized forces applied to the epithelial surface will be transmitted over a wide area of the tissue. In certain diseases, such as pemphigus, where an antibody is erroneously produced that damages these attachments, there is separation of epithelial cell layers so that large clefts (bullous lesions) develop within the epithelium.

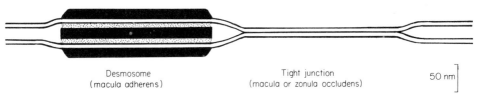

Desmosome
(macula adherens)

Tight junction
(macula or zonula occludens)

50 nm

Fig. 10. Diagram of the two main types of intercellular junction found in oral epithelium.

Tight junctions (Fig. 10) are intercellular junctions in which the adjacent plasma membranes of the epithelial cells are closely apposed so that little or no intercellular space remains. These are rare in oral epithelium as compared to desmosomes and rather than serving as mechanical attachments they may seal off areas of the intercellular space into separate compartments.

The obvious changes accompanying differentiation that are common to all regions of oral epithelium are an increase in cell size and a change in shape (see Fig. 8). These changes are accompanied by the synthesis of more structural protein, the appearance of new organelles and the secretion of additional intercellular material. However, as the basal cells migrate into the prickle cell layer (Fig. 11), slight differences between different regions, such as cell size, become accentuated. The increase in cell size is greater in non-keratinized than in keratinized epithelium, but is not matched by an increase in the number of organelles, so that organelles like the tonofilaments appear less concentrated in the prickle cell layer and remain dispersed through the cell (Fig. 11b). In the prickle cell layer in keratinized epithelium, on the other hand, there is an increase of both synthetic machinery, such as ribosomes, and in the synthesized product, the tonofilaments, which become grouped together into bundles as tonofibrils (Fig. 11a).

In the upper part of the prickle cell layer in both types of epithelia a new organelle makes its appearance—the

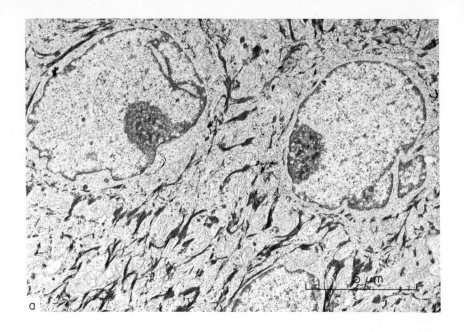

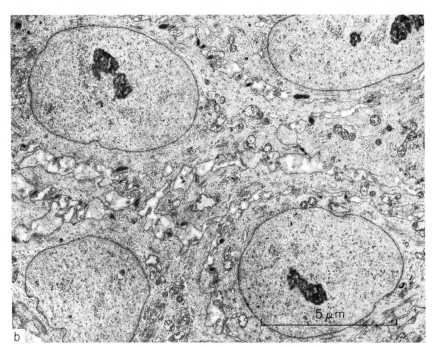

Fig. 11. The ultrastructure of the prickle cell layer. The cells in (a) are from keratinized oral epithelium and contain conspicuous tonofilaments which are gathered together into bundles termed tonofibrils.

In (b), which is taken from non-keratinized oral epithelium, the tonofilaments are sparse although organelles such as mitochondria are abundant.

membrane-coating granule, also called an Odland body or keratinosome. These small membranous structures, some 0·25 μm in length, possibly originate from the Golgi system and are predominantly located in the superficial portion of the cell. The granules have a different morphology in keratinized and non-keratinized epithelium (Fig. 12).

By the time the cells reach the next layer, the granular or intermediate layer, the cells of both keratinized and non-keratinized epithelium have increased in volume and appear more flattened (see Fig. 8). Although all the organelles already mentioned are still present, the cytoplasm is predominantly occupied by the tonofilaments or tonofibrils. The membrane-coating granules, which are gathered along the superficial plasma membrane, appear to fuse with it and discharge their contents into the intercellular space in the upper part of this layer (inset, Fig. 12a). This event seems to be associated with the formation of a barrier to the free movement of substances through the intercellular spaces of the epithelium (see this chapter, section 5). Finally there is a thickening of the internal (cytoplasmic) aspect of the plasma membrane of the cells in this layer.

In keratinizing oral epithelium the characteristic feature of the granular layer is the keratohyalin granule (Figs. 13 and 14a). These are numerous except in the parakeratinized variant where a granular layer may be almost absent. Keratohyalin granules are irregular structures usually 0·5–1 μm in diameter and appear strongly basophilic in the light microscope. Ultrastructurally they are electron dense, surrounded by ribosomes and in close contact with tonofilaments (Fig. 13a). They are thought to form a matrix in which the tonofilaments may become embedded in the keratin layer.

The non-keratinized regions of the oral mucosa do not possess a granular layer, but cells at the same relative level, that is the deeper part of the outer half of the epithelium, show changes which distinguish them from the basal and prickle cells. These include an increase in size, the accumulation of glycogen and occasionally the presence of keratohyalin granules which, although surrounded by ribosomes, differ from their counterparts in keratinized epithelium by appearing more regular and not being associated with tonofilaments (Fig. 13b). The function of keratohyalin granules in non-keratinized

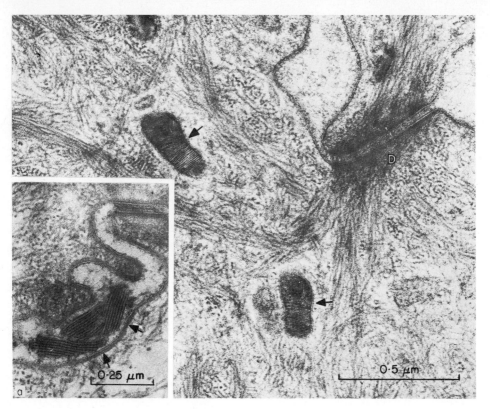

Fig 12. (a) Electron micrograph of a portion of a cell from the granular layer of keratinizing oral epithelium. Two lamellated membrane-coating granules are apparent (arrows). D = desmosome.

Inset: lamellae, presumably derived from membrane coating granules, lying in the intercellular space. Note the thickening on the intracellular aspect of the plasma membrane (arrows).

(b) Electron micrograph of a portion of a cell from the intermediate layer of non-keratinized oral epithelium. A number of 'membrane-coating granules' are present, each with a bounding membrane and central dense core.

PM = plasma membrane.

epithelium is uncertain but they may contribute to the internal thickening of the cell membrane. Superficial to this, there are further gradual changes between successive cell layers of non-keratinized epithelium, although the cells do not appear markedly different from the deeper layer. Scattered tonofilaments are present but are not gathered into bundles, and there is some reduction in the numbers of organelles although many of these, including the nuclei, persist even in the surface layer (Fig. 14b).

The gradual changes in the surface layers of non-keratinized epithelium described above are in contrast to

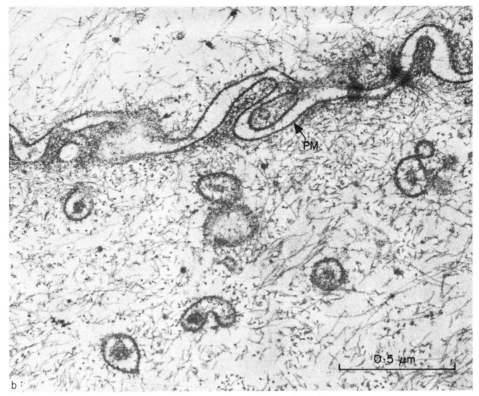

Fig. 12(b)

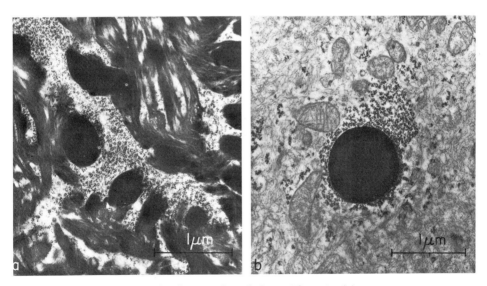

Fig. 13. Keratohyalin granules from oral epithelium. Those in (a) are from keratinized epithelium and are irregular in both size and shape and show a close association with tonofilaments. The granule in (b) is of the type occasionally seen in non-keratinized epithelium and is not associated with tonofilaments.

31

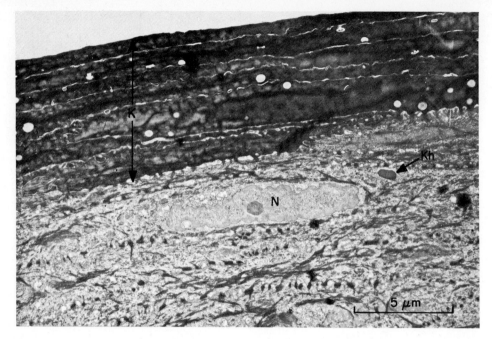

(a)

Fig. 14. Electron micrographs of the superficial cell layers of (a) keratinized and (b) non-keratinized oral epithelium. (a) shows the granular and keratinized layers of gingival epithelium. There is a dramatic change at the junction of these layers, and while a nucleus (N), keratohyalin granule (Kh) and numerous tonofilaments are present in the granular layer, no organelles are apparent in the keratinized layer (K).

(b) is of the superficial layer of buccal epithelium. Tonofilaments are sparse but plump nuclei (N) and other organelles are present in the superficial cells. Note the greater thickness of these cells as compared to the squames of keratinized epithelium (both (a) and (b) are reproduced at similar magnification).

events in ortho-keratinized epithelium (Fig. 14a). In the superficial part of the granular layer dramatic changes take place which include the disappearance of the nuclei and virtually all organelles so that the cells of the keratinized surface layer are filled entirely with tonofilaments. The tonofilaments become surrounded with a matrix, possibly derived from the keratohyalin granules (which are no longer recognizable) and, at the same time, cell size decreases abruptly so the filaments appear tightly packed. The superficial cells, consisting of predominantly dehydrated filamentous material enclosed in a thickened cell envelope, form the hexagonal keratinized squames which are not only mechanically tough but also highly resistant to chemical solvents. They are

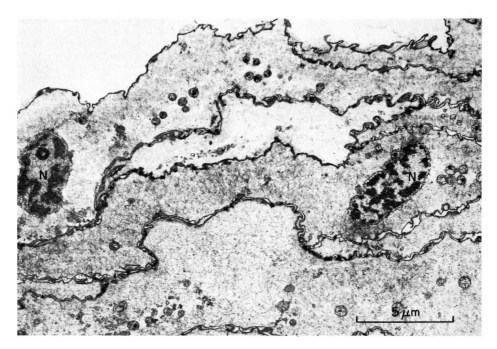

Fig. 14(b)

lost from the surface (desquamated) as a result of abrasion and normal wear and tear (Fig. 15). The keratinized layer is composed of up to 20 rows of squames, which is thicker than that of most areas of epidermis with the exception of the palmar and plantar regions.

In para-keratinization the most obvious feature is the retention of nuclei in the surface squames even though the whole surface layer stains like keratin with eosin and other dyes. Ultrastructurally the cells are packed with filaments, but quite often other organelles as well as the nuclei remain. This suggests that there has been incomplete removal of organelles in the granular layer. Para-keratinization is commonplace in the gingiva (see Fig. 7b) where it may extend to 75% of the area, but it is also occasionally seen in areas of the hard palate.

In some regions of the oral cavity, particularly in the gingiva, there may be some uptake of fluid from the oral cavity into the surface cells of the keratinized layer. This alters their histological staining properties so that with a Mallory trichrome stain for example, these cells stain in the same way as the deeper cells of the epithelium. This appearance has been called 'incomplete' keratinization (or 'incomplete' para-keratinization).

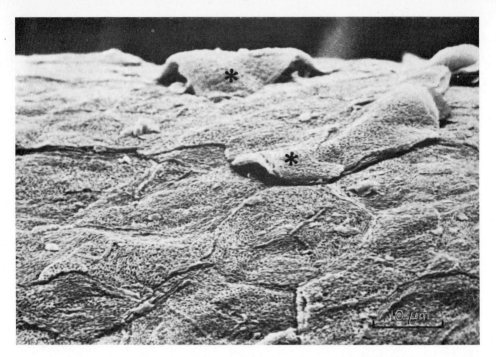

Fig. 15. A scanning electron micrograph of the surface cells of keratinized oral epithelium. The squames have a hexagonal shape and each shows a finely pitted surface pattern. Several squames (asterisks) appear to be desquamating.

It is clear from this account of events leading to the formation of a keratin layer that keratinization is not a single event but represents the sum total of a number of different cellular processes, such as the synthesis and aggregation of tonofilaments, the loss of organelles and the formation of a matrix, all of which occur simultaneously. In the various tissues that we describe as 'keratinized' these different processes may each proceed to different extents to give rise to the differences that distinguish for example, hair from epidermis or para-keratinized oral epithelium from ortho-keratinized epithelium. Even in non-keratinized oral epithelium the potential for keratinization exists in that the synthetic apparatus and numerous tonofilaments are present; this may explain the frequency with which areas of non-keratinized oral mucosa such as the cheek and lip form a keratinized surface when appropriately stimulated. Conversely, the process may not proceed so far under certain conditions, as for example in inflammation, when mucosae that are normally keratinized or para-keratinized, such as the palate and gingiva, show areas of para-keratinization or

34

even non-keratinization. The lamina propria also has an important role to play in determining and controlling the nature of epithelial differentiation, and this is discussed further in Chapter 8, section 2.

3:4 Non-keratinocytes

Histological sections through oral epithelium frequently reveal cells at various levels that differ quite markedly from the rest of the epithelial cells in possessing a clear halo around the nucleus (Fig. 16). Because of this appearance such cells have often been termed 'clear cells', but it is obvious from ultrastructural studies that they can represent any of a variety of cell types such as pigment cells, Langerhans cells, Merkel cells or lympho-cytes which together amount to about 10% of the cell population within epithelium. All these cells differ from the typical epithelial cell in their inability to form keratin

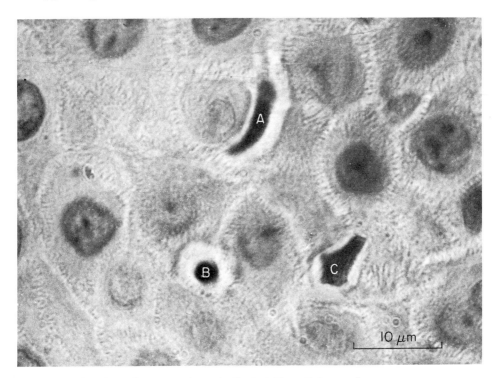

Fig. 16. A histological section through the prickle cell layer of gingival epithelium containing three 'clear cells'. The elongate nuclei of cells A and C suggest they may be Langerhans cells or, possibly, melanocytes. Cell B could be a lymphocyte or merely a cross-section of a cell such as A. Note the appearance of the inter-cellular bridges or 'prickles' between the epithelial cells.

35

Table 2. Characteristics of epithelial 'clear cells'.

Cell type	Level in epithelium	Specific staining reactions	Ultrastructural features
Melanocyte	Basal	DOPA positive; tyrosinase positive; argentaffilic	Dendritic, no desmosomes or tonofilaments; pre-melanosomes and melanosomes present
Langerhans cell	Predominantly supra-basal	Gold chloride positive; osmium iodide positive; ATPase positive	Dendritic, no desmosomes or tonofilaments; characteristic 'Langerhans granule'
Merkel cell	Basal	Probably paS positive	Non-dendritic; sparse desmosomes and tonofilaments; characteristic electron dense vesicles and associated nerve
Lymphocyte	Variable	None	Large circular nucleus; scant cytoplasm with few organelles; no desmosomes or tono-filaments

and all except the Merkel cell lack desmosomes so that the cytoplasm of the cell shrinks against the nucleus during histological processing and produces the typical 'clear' halo. The different types of non-keratinocytes found in oral epithelium are listed in Table 2 together with their histochemical and ultrastructural characteristics, and a more detailed description of each cell is given below.

3:4:1 THE MELANOCYTE AND PIGMENTATION OF ORAL EPITHELIUM

Various names such as melanoblast, melanophore and melanodendrocyte have been applied to the epithelial pigment cell, but the term *melanocyte* has now been universally adopted to describe the dendritic melanin-producing cell that is situated in the basal region of oral epithelium (Fig. 17a). These cells differ from adjacent keratinocytes in many ways—embryologically they are derived from neural crest ectoderm and enter the epithelium from about the eleventh week; once in the epithelium they constitute a self-reproducing population. Ultrastructurally, melanocytes lack the tonofilaments and desmosomes of keratinocytes and synthesize melanin pigment in the form of small organelles called

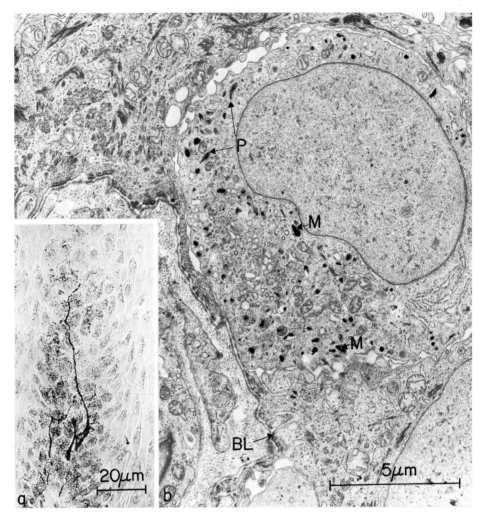

Fig. 17. (a) Light micrograph of a melanocyte in gingival epithelium stained by the Masson-Fontana silver method. The cell body is situated basally although a dendritic process extends well into the prickle cell layer.

(b) Electron micrograph of a melanocyte in buccal epithelium. The cell is situated adjacent to the basal lamina (BL) and pre-melanosomes (P) and melanosomes (M) are present in the cytoplasm.

melanosomes (Fig. 17b). In dark-skinned individuals the melanocytes may be identified in routine haematoxylin and eosin sections by their abundant content of melanosomes which, when grouped together in sufficient numbers, are visible as *melanin granules*. In lightly pigmented persons melanocytes are less active in the production of melanin and may be more easily mistaken for other types of clear cell, although it is possible to apply histochemical tests to identify the presence of enzymes such as tyrosinase or dihydroxyphenyl alanine (DOPA)-oxidase that participate in the synthesis of melanin, or to stain the melanosomes with a silver impregnation technique (argentaffin reaction: see Appendix 1 : 1).

One of the most interesting points about melanin pigmentation is that individuals, regardless of race or degree of pigmentation, all have about the same number of melanocytes in any given region; in the oral mucosa this is approximately one melanocyte to every seven basal epithelial cells. Differences in pigmentation of a given region are thus a function of the activity of the melanocytes in producing melanosomes and in transferring them to the adjacent keratinocytes by a process that has been called 'inoculation'. In this way melanin is introduced into most of the keratinocytes although as the keratinocytes migrate to the surface there is also degradation of the melanosomes so that the superficial cells, except in very heavily pigmented individuals, do not contain pigment.

Cells containing melanin may be seen in the connective tissue beneath normal pigmented oral epithelium; ultrastructural examination of such cells does not reveal any of the characteristics of a melanocyte and it is likely that they represent macrophages containing melanin that must have originated in the epithelium. The term *melanophage* is sometimes applied to these cells (see Fig. 21 and Chapter 4, section 1).

There is a direct relationship between the degree of melanin pigmentation seen in the skin and that found in the oral mucosa, where the most commonly pigmented regions are the lips, the gingiva, the buccal mucosa and the soft palate. However the degree of pigmentation varies considerably with race and light skinned caucasoids rarely show any oral pigmentation at all. Apart from melanin, factors such as the thickness of the epithelium, the degree of keratinization, the vascularity of the underlying connective tissue and the relative amounts of reduced or oxidized haemoglobin and the presence of subcutaneous fat all contribute to the colour of the oral mucosa. Unlike the epidermis, the oral epithelium is non-keratinized in many areas, possesses a thin keratin layer in other areas and overlays an extensively vascularized connective tissue so the resulting coloration is a brighter red than is seen anywhere in the skin. Apart from these features, which represent what may be termed endogenous pigmentation, there is also exogenous pigmentation, in which foreign material such as heavy metals or carbon, having been introduced either systemically or locally into the body, produce coloration of the oral tissues. A frequent example of this is the presence beneath the gingival epithelium of particles of dental amalgam causing patches of bluish-grey pigmentation known as amalgam tattoo. In histological sections it is not difficult to distinguish this exogenous pigmentation from melanin, particularly if special stains are applied.

3:4:2 THE LANGERHANS CELL

This cell was first described by Paul Langerhans in 1868 during a study of sections of human epidermis impregnated with gold chloride. Positively staining dendritic cells were present in the upper layers of the epidermis, a distribution that led to their being termed 'high level' clear cells, although it is now known that they can also be found in the deeper layers. More recently these cells have been found in the oral epithelium. Like the melanocyte, Langerhans cells are dendritic and lack tonofilaments and desmosomes, but they do not synthesize melanin. Instead they contain a characteristic rod-shaped body called the Langerhans granule (Fig. 18). Langerhans cells may be demonstrated histologically by metal impregnation (see inset, Fig. 18), but these methods are unreliable and the most consistent identification seems to be obtained by carrying out a histochemical reaction for the enzyme adenosine triphosphatase (ATPase) which stains the Langerhans cell membrane preferentially.

Langerhans cells appear in developing epithelium before, or at the same time as, the melanocyte but they do not seem to be derived from the neural crest and their origin is unknown. Their function in epidermis and oral epithelium is debatable and they have been variously described as neural elements, as degenerate melanocytes, as intra-epithelial macrophages and as regulatory cells, controlling epithelial cell division and differentiation. There is no convincing evidence for any of these roles although recently it has been shown that in skin they may be involved in the uptake and processing of

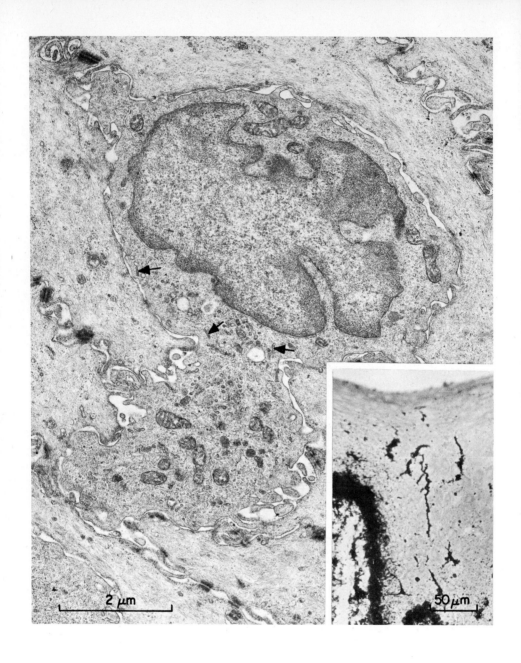

Fig. 18. Electron micrograph of a Langerhans cell in buccal epithelium. The cell is dendritic with a deeply indented nucleus and a number of characteristic rod-shaped Langerhans granules (arrows) may be seen.

Inset: A histological section through gingival epithelium that has been impregnated with gold chloride. This stains the basement membrane region and also several 'high level' dendritic cells which may be Langerhans cells (see text).

40

antigenic materials in contact allergic reactions; this would place them in the macrophage category.

3:4:3 THE MERKEL CELL AND INTRA-EPITHELIAL NERVES

Merkel cells appear histologically as 'clear cells' situated basally in oral epithelium, although they do not have the dendritic shape characteristic of the melanocyte and Langerhans cell. They were described by Merkel in 1875 in the gingiva and have since been reported in other regions of oral epithelium as well as in epidermis. Ultrastructurally (Fig. 19) the Merkel cell has sparse tonofilaments, occasional desmosome attachments to adjacent keratinocytes and a nerve fibre is often seen to be associated with the cell. A characteristic feature is the small dense membrane-bounded granules that may liberate a transmitter substance across the synapse-like cleft between the cell and the adjacent nerve. This arrangement fits in with the concept of the Merkel cell as a sensory

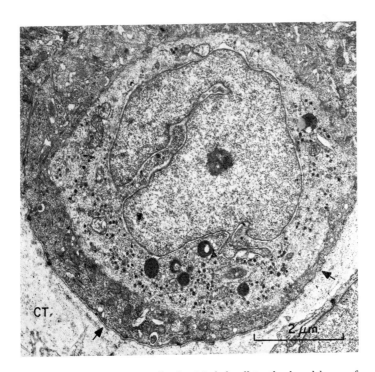

Fig. 19. Electron micrograph of a Merkel cell in the basal layer of oral epithelium (the basal lamina is indicated by arrows). The cytoplasm is much lighter than that of adjacent keratinocytes and contains numerous small dense granules. CT = connective tissue.

41

cell responding to touch. It is of interest that Merkel cells have been identified in biopsies of aphthous ulcers where it was suggested that the release of catecholamines from the small granules might contribute to the necrosis of the epithelial-connective tissue region which accompanies the development of aphthous ulceration.

Intra-epithelial nerves frequently have been demonstrated in oral epithelium, particularly in the gingiva. These nerves are never associated with specialized investing cells such as Schwann cells, but run between the epithelial cells which often ensheath or completely enclose the nerve to form a mesaxon. The nerves terminate in the middle or upper epithelial layers as simple endings (see Chapter 4, section 5).

3:4:4 OTHER NON-KERATINOCYTES

Lymphocytes may be seen in many regions of oral epithelium from persons with clinically normal oral mucosa, while the epithelium applied to the tooth (junctional and oral sulcular epithelium, see Chapter 6, section 4) is often infiltrated with both mononuclear cells and neutrophilic granulocytes. Mast cells have also been demonstrated in gingival epithelium. All these cells are immigrants in the epithelium, usually for a short period of time and do not have the status of a self-perpetuating population such as the other non-keratinocytes we have considered. Nevertheless it is rare to see a section of oral epithelium without some inflammatory cells and their presence must be considered commonplace.

3:5 The permeability of oral epithelium

From a structural point of view the oral epithelium is an impressive barrier, consisting of a specialized surface layer beneath which are several layers of closely apposed cells separated from the lamina propria by a continuous basement membrane capable of restraining all but the smallest particles. The connective tissue, on the other hand, only limits the passage of very large molecules and plays little part in the barrier function of the mucosa as a whole.

While the superficial layer of intact oral epithelium prevents the entry of relatively large objects, such as micro-organisms, the mechanism by which the diffusion

42

of molecules and ions is controlled is less clear, since there are two potential routes across the epithelium for such substances depending on their size and chemical nature. One route involves passing through the inter-cellular spaces between the cells, the other involves entering into and crossing the cells themselves. The most important property that determines whether a given substance will pass rapidly across the oral mucosa seems to be its relative solubility between lipid and water. Those substances with a high solubility in lipid traverse the oral mucosa most easily, possibly by moving along, or across, the lipid rich plasma membranes of the epithelial cells, while water soluble substances and ions probably move through the intercellular spaces between the cells.

Because of the apparent ease with which drugs can be absorbed orally, the mucosa is often regarded as a highly permeable membrane, this property being ascribed particularly to the areas of non-keratinized epithelium present in the oral cavity. However experiments using tracer substances detectable in the electron microscope have shown that an intercellular barrier exists which limits the movement of certain substances between the cells of both keratinized and non-keratinized regions of oral mucosa. This barrier is similar to that found in the epidermis and is situated between cells in the keratinized or superficial layer of the epithelium and seems to arise as a result of the membrane-coating granules being dis-charged into the intercellular space (see this chapter, section 3). There is little known about the permeability of keratinized or non-keratinized epithelium to those substances which may pass through the cells.

One region of the oral cavity that is of considerable importance in the context of permeability is the junc-tional epithelium where the oral epithelium meets the erupted tooth surface (see Chapter 6, section 4, for a description of the structure of this area). The epithelium at this site has been shown to be permeable to a wide range of different substances including bacterial toxins and enzymes which, once they have gained access to the underlying tissues can readily initiate inflammation which leads to gingivitis and periodontal disease. Whether the permeability of this region is due to intrinsic differences in the structure of the junctional epithelium or to damage resulting from dental plaque is uncertain.

43

Further reading

ALVARES O.F. & MEYER J. (1971) Variable features and regional differences in oral epithelium. In *Current Concepts of the Histology of Oral Mucosa* (edited by Squier, C.A. and Meyer, J.) 97–113, Charles C. Thomas, Springfield, Ill.

PARAKKAL P.F. & ALEXANDER N.J. (1972) *Keratinization: a survey of vertebrate epithelia.* Academic Press, New York.

SKOUGAARD M. (1970) Cell renewal with special reference to the gingival epithelium. *Advances Oral Biol.* **4**, 261–288.

SQUIER C.A. & JOHNSON N.W. (1975) The permeability of oral mucosa. *Brit. Med. Bull* **31**, 169–175.

44

CHAPTER 4
THE CONNECTIVE TISSUE

Despite the importance of the epithelium as a barrier layer, many of the mechanical properties of oral mucosa depend on the underlying connective tissue (the lamina propria or corium) which also attaches the epithelium to deeper structures.

The bulk of the connective tissue consists of a collagen fibre network, the organization of which determines the mechanical stability and the resistance to deformation and extensibility of the tissue. Present in smaller amounts are elastic fibres, which serve to restore deformed collagen to its relaxed state and reticulin fibres which enmesh bundles of collagen fibres and are predominant in the basement membrane region. This fibre system is permeated by a highly hydrated matrix or ground substance composed of carbohydrate—protein complexes (see Appendix 2) in which are situated the cells responsible for secreting and maintaining both fibres and matrix together with those cells concerned with defence reactions. The lamina propria is penetrated by elements of the nervous system, sensory branches of which enter the epithelium, and by the blood vascular and lymphatic systems which run close to, but never enter, the epithelium. There are considerable differences in the relative proportions of each of these elements, particularly the fibres, in different regions of the oral mucosa and this is discussed more fully in Chapter 6. What follows here is a general account applicable to all regions.

Morphologically, the lamina propria may be divided into two layers, a superficial zone of loose connective tissue adjacent to the epithelium and surrounding the epithelial ridges—the *papillary layer*, and a deeper zone of denser connective tissue called, because of the net-like appearance of its fibre bundles, the *reticular layer* (see Fig. 3). The differences between these layers are not clear cut and it is the relative concentration and arrangement of fibres rather than any absolute differences that enable these regions to be distinguished. The papillary layer contains predominantly fine collagen fibres arranged as a loose open network. In the region of the basement membrane these fibres are associated with reticulin fibres, while at the junction with the subjacent reticular layer they merge into thicker collagen bundles. Where appendages are present the papillary layer is reflected deeply so as to surround them. In the reticular layer the collagen fibres are coarser and closely packed. They are often arranged in laminae in the plane of the surface (the horizontal plane), while in the vertical plane most are aligned in the direction of minimum extensibility.

In this chapter the various components of the lamina propria, the cells, fibres and ground substance, blood vessels and nerves, are described. From a structural point of view it must be remembered that the various elements of the connective tissue of oral mucosa do not differ greatly from those of skin or from connective tissues elsewhere in the body; functionally there are sometimes greater differences, as for example, in the circulatory system, which participates in temperature regulation in the skin but probably not in the oral mucosa.

4:1 The cells of the connective tissue

From a functional point of view the connective tissue of oral mucosa must contain cells responsible for the synthesis and maintenance of its structure and for the defence of the tissue and the organism. In the former group are cells synthesizing and secreting fibres and ground substance—the fibroblasts or fibrocytes and adipose or fat cells concerned with the synthesis and storage of fat. Cells with a role in defence are the macrophage or histiocyte, the mast cell and variable numbers of 'inflammatory cells' derived from circulating leuco-

46

cytes. In addition there are undifferentiated mesenchymal cells which because of their dormancy cannot be assigned to one of the above functional groups, and the constituent cells of vascular and lymphatic channels and of neural elements.

All these cells are fundamentally the same as their counterparts in connective tissue elsewhere, differing only in numbers and degree of function. Within the oral mucosa there are marked differences between both the absolute and relative numbers of each cell from area to area, reflecting different functions of various regions. Because structure and function are so closely related, it should be realized that the appearance of any cell will depend not only on the major functional group to which it belongs but also on its level of activity at the moment of tissue fixation. The characteristics of the main connective tissue cells are set out below and summarized in Table 3.

4:1:1 FIBROBLASTS AND FIBROCYTES

In the light microscope the fibroblast appears as an elongated fusiform or stellate cell with an elliptical nucleus containing several prominent nucleoli; the cells are aligned parallel to the neighbouring collagen fibre bundles (Fig. 20a). Quiescent cells, sometimes termed fibrocytes, have relatively little cytoplasm which may be difficult to detect in routine preparations.

The ultrastructure of a fibroblast (Fig. 20b) is that of the typical secretory cell, with abundant rough endoplasmic reticulum, a well developed Golgi apparatus and numerous membrane-bound vesicles located near the cell boundaries. Current opinion is that newly synthesized collagen sub-units aggregate within the cisternae of the endoplasmic reticulum and probably within Golgi vesicles from which they are secreted after fusion with the plasma membrane. Further aggregation to typically banded fibrils (see inset, Fig. 20b and Fig. 23) takes place extracellularly in association with the protein-polysaccharide complexes of the ground substance also secreted by the fibroblast (see this chapter, section 2). Mature collagen fibrils are frequently seen in close apposition to the plasma membrane and shrinkage of tissue components during processing for electron microscopy may exaggerate the space between collagen and the fibroblast.

47

Table 3. Main cell types found in the lamina propria of oral mucosa.

Cell type	Origin	Morphological and staining characteristics
Fibroblast	Mesenchymal cell	Stellate, or elongated cell, palely haematoxophilic with prominent nucleoli
Histiocyte	Mesenchymal cell	Spindle shaped or stellate cell, often darkly staining nucleus
Monocyte	Bone marrow via circulation	Round cell with darkly staining kidney-shaped nucleus and moderate amount of cytoplasm
Macrophage	Histiocyte or monocyte	Round cell with palely staining nucleus and abundant, often 'foamy', cytoplasm
Polymorphonuclear leucocyte (neutrophil)	Bone marrow via circulation	Round cell with characteristic lobed nucleus
Mast cell	Mesenchymal cell	Round or oval shaped cell with basophilic granules which stain meta-chromatically
Lymphocyte	Bone marrow and lymph nodes via circulation	Round cell with darkly staining nucleus and little cytoplasm
Plasma cell	B lymphocytes from bone marrow and lymph nodes via circulation	Cartwheel nucleus. Intensely pyronino-philic cytoplasm
Endothelial cell	Mesenchymal cell	Non-specific

4:1:2 MACROPHAGES AND HISTIOCYTES

Macrophages are chiefly characterized by their potential for extensive phagocytosis. Their function is to ingest and break down micro-organisms, foreign material and fragments of damaged tissue following injury. In addition they have important immune functions involving the recognition, ingestion and 'processing' of antigen for subsequent presentation to cells of the lympoid series in which antibody synthesis takes place.

There is a wide variety of morphological types

Ultrastructural features	Function	Distribution
Abundant rough endo-plasmic reticulum	Secretion of fibres and ground substance	Throughout lamina propria
Lysosomal vesicles	Precursor of functional macrophage	Throughout lamina propria
Lysosomes and phagocytic vesicles. Few free ribosomes, some endoplasmic reticulum. Prominent Golgi apparatus	Phagocytic cell. Precursor of macrophage	Areas of inflammation
Lysosomes and phagocytic vesicles	Phagocytosis including antigen processing	Areas of chronic inflammation
Lysosomes and specific granules	Phagocytosis and cell-killing	Areas of acute inflammation within lamina propria. May be present in epithelium
Characteristic granules	Secretion of certain inflammatory mediators (histamine, heparin)	Throughout lamina propria, often sub-epithelial
Scant cytoplasm with a few mitochondria. Little or no endoplasmic reticulum, large number of free ribosomes	Participates in humoral and cell-mediated immune response	Areas of acute and chronic inflammation
Abundant rough endo-plasmic reticulum	Synthesis of immuno-globulins	Areas of chronic inflam-mation, often perivascularly
Normally associated with a basal lamina and contains numerous pinocytotic vesicles	Lining cell of blood and lymphatic channels	Lining vascular channels throughout lamina propria

amongst cells of the macrophage series. Once the cytoplasm contains large amounts of ingested material identification is easy, particularly if this material is pigmented like haemosiderin or distinctive in shape, like bacteria or fungi. Such cells are usually large (up to 50 μm or more in diameter) and spherical with a dense, sometimes kidney-shaped, nucleus compressed to one side. Identification in the electron microscope (Fig. 21) is more straightforward because of the large number of phagocytic vacuoles; the cell membrane is often convoluted and material may sometimes be seen apparently

49

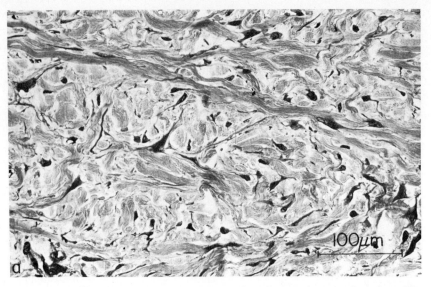

Fig. 20. (a) Lamina propria of oral mucosa stained with Held's molybdic acid–haematoxylin to demonstrate cell cytoplasm. Most of the cells are fibroblasts and are elongate or stellate with long cytoplasmic processes. Processes of cells whose bodies are not in the plane of section are aligned along and between collagen fibre bundles.

(b) Electron micrograph of a fibroblast in gingiva. The cell body is stellate and contains the nucleus (N) numerous mitochondria (M) a Golgi apparatus (G) and a rough-surfaced endoplasmic reticulum (ER) with dilated cisternae containing finely granular material. Portions of several narrow cytoplasmic processes can be seen in close association with transversely sectioned collagen fibrils.

Inset: longitudinally sectioned collagen fibrils revealing the characteristic cross-banding.

being phagocytosed. Quiescent histiocytes are more difficult to identify and closely resemble fibroblasts in light microscope preparations. They are frequently complex stellate cells with long branching cytoplasmic extensions and the nucleus is usually smaller and denser than that of the fibroblast, with inconspicuous nucleoli.

Normal non-inflamed tissue contains 'fixed' or stationary cells, the histiocytes, which are related to other 'fixed' phagocytes of the reticulo-endothelial system. In inflamed mucosa, monocytes enter the tissue from the blood and differentiate to form macrophages. Thus both monocytes and macrophages in various states of differentiation will be found in the lamina propria if inflammation is present. Functional macrophages originating in this way are indistinguishable from those derived from the histiocytes normally present.

50

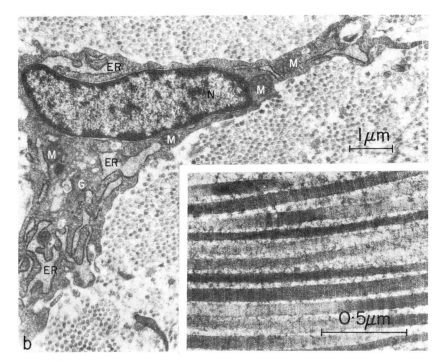

Fig. 20(b)

Melanophages and siderophages. Macrophages in the lamina propria may ingest melanin granules from the epithelium and are common in pigmented oral mucosa. Such melanophages contain mature melanin granules (Fig. 21) undergoing degradation and are not capable of melanin synthesis.

Haemosiderin, derived from red blood cells spilled into the tissue following vascular injury, is taken up by cells of the macrophage line and ultimately degraded *in situ* or carried away to other parts of the reticulo-endothelial system. These cells are termed siderophages and may persist for many weeks at the site of injured or inflamed mucosa when other signs of inflammation have faded. Iron containing pigments can be differentiated readily from melanin and other pigments in tissues by the use of special stains.

4:1:3 MAST CELLS

Mast cells were originally described by Ehrlich in 1877 on the basis of the highly distinctive metachromatic granules filling their cytoplasm. The metachromasia of

51

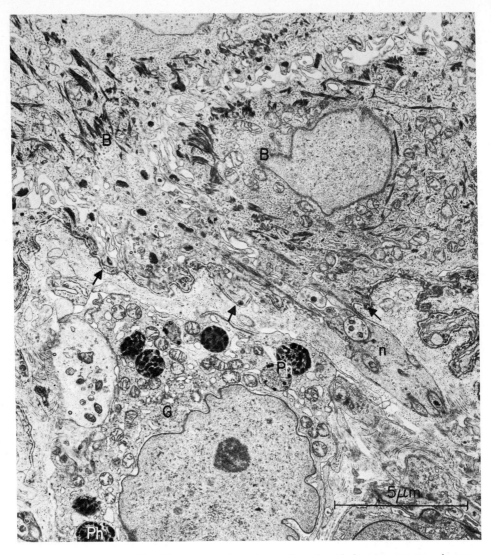

Fig. 21. A macrophage beneath oral epithelium containing electron-dense melanosomes within phagosomes (Ph). Numerous mito-chondria and Golgi vesicles (G) are visible and the plasma membrane is thrown into a number of microvilli. This cell can be termed a melanophage. A non-myelinated nerve (n) penetrates the basal lamina (arrows) and passes into the epithelium between the basal cells (B).

these granules is due to the presence of the proteoglycan heparin (see Appendix 2) and in addition the granules contain histamine. These substances with their anti-coagulent and vaso-active properties may play a role in maintaining normal tissue and vascular homeostasis; they are particularly important in inflammation.

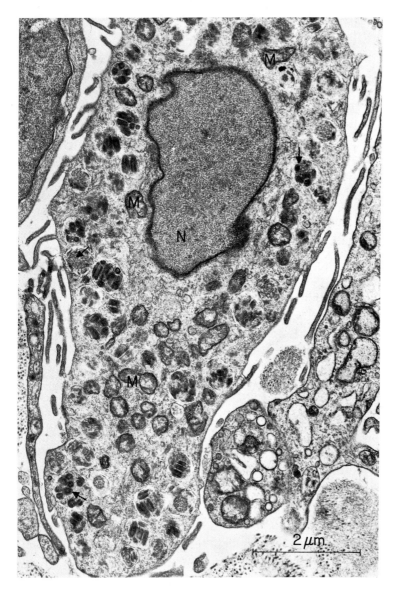

Fig. 22. Mast cell. Numerous long microvilli project from the cell surface and the cytoplasm contains many characteristic granules (arrows). N = nucleus, M = mitochondrion.

The mast cell is a large spherical or elliptical cell, up to 40 μm in length, with a relatively small centrally placed nucleus. The cytoplasm stains fairly intensely with both acidic and basic dyes and dyes such as toluidine blue, methylene blue or thionine are converted to a purple metachromatic hue within the granules. In the electron microscope (Fig. 22) these cells are highly distinctive, the two main distinguishing features being the presence of numerous micro-villi projecting from the plasma membrane and large numbers of characteristic cytoplasmic granules.

Whilst the granules of tissue mast cells are very similar to those of the circulating blood basophils there is no conclusive evidence that they are derived from these granulocytes. Mast cells in oral mucosa tend to be distributed in perivascular and perineural locations; they are particularly common in the lamina propria of lining mucosa and in the tongue. Occasionally, they are present in normal oral epithelium.

4:1:4 LYMPHOCYTES AND PLASMA CELLS

Lymphocytes of various types and their progeny are the essential immunocompetent cells of the body and there has been a great increase in knowledge of their structure and functions in the past decade. A comprehensive survey of this is outside the scope of the present volume because we are primarily concerned with normal mucosa. Lymphocytes and plasma cells are normally only present in significant numbers in this tissue as part of a disease process or defence reaction but as this is so common in oral mucosa, particularly in the gingiva, some account of their structure is necessary. Furthermore, lymphocyte aggregations are a normal component of certain regions of the oral mucosa, such as the lingual tonsils.

The small lymphocyte. This cell is present in circulating blood and lymph, in lymph nodes and spleen, in the thymus and in the lymphoid tissue associated with the gastro-intestinal tract. It is, at the light microscope level, a simple round cell approximately 6–10 μm in diameter with a dense nucleus and minimal cytoplasm. In the electron microscope the cytoplasm is seen to contain a few mitochondria, and scattered ribosomes but little rough endoplasmic reticulum. Cells of this appearance are present in inflammatory foci in oral mucosa, and in small numbers in both the connective tissue and epithelium of apparently healthy tissue.

Small lymphocytes fall into two major functional groups indistinguishable by routine microscopy. T lymphocytes are derived from or processed by and dependent on the thymus for their function (T = thymus), whilst

54

the B lymphocyte is dependent on certain peripheral lymphoid tissue. This tissue is the bursa of Fabricius in birds (B = bursa), and in man is probably represented by gastro-intestinal lymphoid tissue such as Peyer's patches and possibly also the tonsils.

T lymphocytes are responsible for cell mediated immunity i.e. processes such as graft rejection and delayed hypersensitivity; many diseases of the oral mucosa have a large cell mediated immune component. B lymphocytes are responsible for the second arm of the immune response—humoral immunity. When stimulated by specific antigen a clone of B lymphocytes will proliferate and differentiate into plasma cells which synthesize and secrete immunoglobulin.

Plasma cells. The mature plasma cell is readily identifiable as a round or oval cell up to 20 μm in diameter with an eccentrically placed nucleus containing discrete chromatin granules arranged in the so-called 'clockface' or 'cart-wheel' pattern. The plentiful cytoplasm is basophilic and intensely pyroninophilic (see Table, Appendix 1) due to the extensive RNA content. Electron microscopy reveals an abundant rough endoplasmic reticulum on which antibody synthesis takes place.

Plasma cells are frequently seen in areas of inflammation in the oral mucosa, particularly in chronic gingivitis and in the lingual tonsils. Various stages in the maturation of these cells can be recognized and in long standing foci of chronic inflammation lightly eosinophilic spherical aggregates of immunoglobulin, the so-called Russell bodies, may be seen both within and between plasma cells.

4:1:5 GRANULOCYTES

Granular leucocytes, comprising neutrophils, eosinophils and basophils, are components of certain types of inflammatory reaction in oral mucosa as elsewhere in the body. Neutrophils are most commonly encountered and may occasionally be found in the lamina propria of apparently healthy tissue. They are almost always present in significant numbers in gingival exudate, even in the absence of clinical gingivitis and in gingiva are mostly observed within blood vessels, in the process of traversing vessel walls, or within the sulcular and junctional epithelium (see Chapter 6, section 4).

Under the light microscope these cells have a highly characteristic morphology, possessing a lobulated nucleus and a cytoplasm filled with fine granules. Ultra-structurally, the lobed nucleus may appear in section as separate nuclei; the cytoplasm contains two types of granules, specific granules which contain alkaline phosphatase and collagenase and the azurophilic granules which contain peroxidase and a variety of hydrolytic enzymes and are similar to lysosomes.

4:2 Fibre types of the connective tissue

4:2:1 COLLAGEN FIBRES

Gross structure. Branching bundles of collagen fibres can be seen in the connective tissue of skin and oral mucosa by light microscopy (see Fig. 20a). The fibres are palely eosinophilic in a standard haematoxylin and eosin preparation but are more readily observed in material stained by Van Gieson's picrofuchsin method, when the collagen fibres appear red against a green background.

Individual collagen fibres are approximately 200 nm in diameter and do not branch, being composed of smaller non-branching fibrils visible only at the electron microscope level. Such fibrils vary greatly in diameter, but it is only in those with a diameter greater than 10 nm that the characteristic banding pattern, repeating every 64 nm, can be observed (inset, Fig. 20).

Molecular structure. Collagen is a glycoprotein (see Appendix 2) containing approximately 0·3–0·5% by weight of carbohydrate. Whilst the carbohydrate portion comprises the simple hexose sugars galactose and glucose (which is rarely found in glycoproteins), the protein portion is characterized by a high glycine content and the presence of two unusual amino acids—hydroxyproline and hydroxylysine. Indeed the presence of hydroxyproline forms the basis of standard biochemical assays of collagen.

The primary structure of collagen is a polypeptide chain, synthesized on the rough endoplasmic reticulum of fibroblasts, and in which every third amino acid residue is glycine. Proline and lysine are at this stage present but in their unhydroxylated forms. This polypeptide chain stabilizes itself in the form of an alpha-

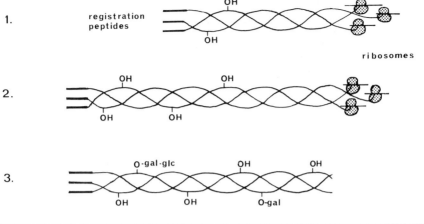

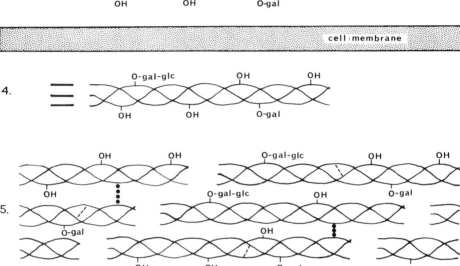

Fig. 23. Stages of collagen synthesis. The synthesis, hydroxylation and glycosylation (stages 1–3) all take place intra-cellularly. The pro-collagen then leaves the cells, the registration peptides are removed (4) and there is alignment and cross-linking to form the collagen fibrils (5). The two types of cross-linking, intra-molecular and inter-molecular, are represented by broken lines and dotted lines respectively.

helix and three such chains align, aided by 'registration' peptides located in the N terminals of the chains, and intertwine to form a coiled-coil in which the individual alpha-chains are held together by hydrogen bonding (Fig. 23 (1)). This form of collagen, which has sometimes been referred to as protocollagen, undergoes hydroxylation and glycosylation to become pro-collagen. The process of hydroxylation (Fig. 23 (1)–(3)) is enzymatic and requires vitamin C, ferrous ions, α-ketoglutarate and molecular oxygen. This process begins

57

during translation but is not completed until after the molecule has been released from the poly-ribosomes. Glycosylation (Fig. 23 (3)) involves the addition of galactose to specific hydroxylysine residues followed, at a variable number of these sites, by glucose, and this is thought to occur in the Golgi region of the cell or at the plasma membrane.

Procollagen is extruded from the cell and the registration peptides cleaved from the rest of the molecule by the enzyme pro-collagen peptidase (Fig. 23 (4)). This form of collagen has in the past been referred to as tropocollagen although this term is now rarely used. It is these extracellular collagen molecules, now approximately 290 nm long, that align themselves in a parallel arrangement to form the collagen fibrils visible in the electron microscope, as described above (Fig. 23 (5)). This alignment of collagen involves a one quarter overlap of molecules and it is this overlap or 'stagger' which is believed to give rise to the observed 64 nm periodicity. The finer cross banding seen within the main 64 nm bands can be accounted for in part by irregular repeating units within the collagen alpha-chains. The fibrils thus formed are stabilized by intra-molecular and more importantly by inter-molecular covalent cross linking, the extent of which increases with age. Thus whilst young collagen can be partly solubilized in cold salt solutions, as it gets older it requires acids to dissolve it, and eventually becomes totally insoluble.

In recent years it has become apparent that site differences exist between collagens. Thus at least four distinct types of collagen are now recognized, viz. I skin and bone, II cartilage, III basement membrane, and IV fetal, which is found in young skin but rapidly disappears with age. These differences relate to the amino acid sequence in the three alpha chains. Studies on oral mucosa have shown that the collagen of gingiva and palate is predominantly type I collagen.

Apart from these differences, there can be post translational differences in collagens for example in the amount of cross-linking or number of glucosyl residues attached to galactosyl residues. These differences result in collagen with different properties and it is for these reasons that the collagen of skin and presumably oral mucosa, is more soluble, less densely packed and more hydrated than that of bone.

4:2:2 RETICULIN FIBRES

To the light microscopist, reticulin denotes those fibres which are characteristically argyrophilic, i.e. they have the capacity to adsorb metallic silver when treated with alkaline solutions of reducible silver salts. At the electron microscope level, however, these fibres are indistinguishable from collagen, and consist essentially of collagen fibrils coated with ground substance and organized into fibres. There do, however, appear to be two types of reticulin fibres—a fine branching network of fibres about 1 nm in diameter most obvious in developing embryonic connective tissue but also present in the mature connective tissues of skin and gingiva around the mature collagen fibres, and the thicker, wavy, unbranched, fibres which may represent an immature form of collagen coated with ground substances. It appears unlikely that the two forms of reticulin viz. the fine network of branching fibres and the thicker, unbranched wavy form, are related but rather that these two components are synthesized independently by fibroblasts and that only the thicker fibres develop into mature collagen fibres.

4:2:3 ELASTIC FIBRES

Elastic fibres are found in most regions of the oral mucosa, being best represented in the highly deformable lining mucosa. Unlike collagen fibres, elastic fibres branch and anastomose and run singly rather than in bundles. They can be recognized easily in the light microscope by their selective staining with, for example, Orcein or Weigert's resorcin-fuchsin stain. (Fig. 29b shows elastic fibres in alveolar mucosa stained by Hart's elastic stain, which is a modification of Weigert's method). Ultrastructurally, mature elastic fibres appear to comprise a central granular core area surrounded by an envelope of hollow fibrils (microfibrils) each 10–20 nm in diameter. The fibrils display no periodicity although they occasionally have a beaded appearance.

During morphogenesis the first formed elastic fibres consist of aggregates of microfibrils only. With increased maturation the amorphous, granular material is progressively laid down, predominantly within bundles of microfibrils until at maturity it accounts for 90% of the fibre. Although at this stage the microfibrils envelop the granular material, some of them can also be seen embedded within this material. It is said that in aged fibres the peripheral fibrils disappear, presumably because of incorporation within subsequently formed granular material.

Relatively little is known of the method of synthesis or the molecular structure of elastic fibres. It appears that the microfibrils consist of a glycoprotein, the protein component being rich in cysteine and polar amino acids but lacking hydroxyproline and hydroxylysine. The central granular region comprises elastin, a protein characterized by its high glycine content and the presence of two unusual amino acid residues, desmosine and isodesmosine. The latter are synthesized from lysine residues after the polypeptide chain has been assembled, and form strong bridges or cross links between adjacent polypeptide chains. An early form of elastin containing neither desmosine nor isodesmosine residues but with a correspondingly increased lysine content has been identified; this is tropoelastin and is analagous to protocollagen. Subsequent formation of these residues gives a highly cross-linked elastin molecule of remarkable insolubility.

4:2:4 OXYTALAN FIBRES

Oxytalan fibres have been described in the periodontal membrane of man, monkeys, rats, guinea pigs and mice but they have not been conclusively demonstrated in other sites in the body nor have they been found in the periodontal membranes of other species such as dogs, swine and cattle where analagously distributed fibres have all the characteristics of elastic fibres. Indeed oxytalan fibres can be both stained by elastic stains and digested by elastase but only after prior oxidation of the tissue with, for example, per-acetic acid. In this way oxytalan resembles immature elastic fibres which cannot be stained with elastic stains without prior oxidation. Although in the light microscope oxytalan and elastic fibres cannot be distinguished, there is some evidence that there may be slight ultrastructural differences. Oxytalan, like elastic fibres, appears to comprise fibrillar and amorphous elements, but it is said that in mature oxytalan the fibrils are more obvious. There is clearly a need to investigate the differences between these fibres in greater depth; at the moment it is only possible to say that oxytalan appears to resemble immature elastic fibres in much the same way as one type of reticulin resembles immature collagen.

4:3 The ground substance of the connective tissue

The ground substance or matrix of loose connective tissue is a heterogeneous colloidal complex which embeds all other connective tissue components. As no structural features are apparent at the light or electron microscope levels, it has frequently been described as amorphous, although there is now evidence indicating that it has a high degree of macromolecular organization.

The structural components of ground substance consist essentially of carbohydrate-protein complexes which are permeated by tissue fluids. The latter contain plasma proteins, vitamins, hormones, enzymes, electrolytes and metabolic substrates. The matrix is in a continual state of flux, its exact composition being dependent to a large extent on the general metabolic state of the surrounding cells and of the organism as a whole.

4:3:1 CARBOHYDRATE-PROTEIN COMPLEXES ('MUCOSUBSTANCES')

The 'amorphous' ground substance of connective tissue was thought originally to belong to a chemically ill-defined group of substances called mucoids. It subsequently became apparent that this intercellular and interfibrillar substance consisted chiefly of carbohydrate in most cases covalently linked with varying amounts of protein. Terminology has been, and still is, confused although it is now common to divide carbohydrate-protein complexes or mucosubstances into two main groups, proteoglycans and glycoproteins. The staining properties and structure of these two groups of substances are dealt with more fully in Appendix 2.

There are two prominent proteoglycans in the loose connective tissue of skin and oral mucosa, one containing hyaluronic acid, the other chondroitin sulphate B (also known as dermatan sulphate). These molecules contain very long polysaccharide chains bearing negatively charged groups and thus occupy a relatively large amount of space or 'domain'. Hyaluronic acid is more flexible than the comparatively rigid chondroitin sulphate B chains and may be more important than the latter in controlling the passage of molecules through the tissue and the capacity of the tissue to hold water.

The glycoproteins present in the ground substance of skin and oral mucosa are extremely heterogeneous and have not been classified in as much detail as proteoglycans.

4:4 The vascular system of the oral mucosa

Although the thickness of the oral epithelium may exceed 500 μm in some areas, the tissue is avascular and depends for its metabolic requirements on the blood supply to the lamina propria beneath. In general, the oral mucosa has a more concentrated network of vessels than is present in the skin and this is one reason for its greater coloration. As in skin, the blood supply to the oral mucosa is probably in excess of local metabolic requirements but it seems unlikely that here the vascular system has a role to play in thermal regulation. However wound healing in oral mucosa is faster than in skin, and this may reflect a better blood flow. Another feature which has been attributed to the richness of the vascularity is the frequency of mitoses in the overlying epithelium; while there is some data for such an association, the evidence is slender.

The blood supply of the oral cavity is derived predominantly from branches of the external carotid artery, in particular the lingual, facial and maxillary arteries. Arteries supplying the oral mucosa run beneath the mucosa, except where there is a periosteum present, when they run in the deeper part of the lamina propria. They give off progressively smaller branches within the lamina propria; the arterioles, terminal arterioles, metarterioles and capillaries; the most profuse branching occurs between the metarterioles and capillaries. The capillaries form networks of anastamosing branches, one capillary network lying immediately beneath the reticular layer and corresponding to the rete cutaneum of the skin while that forming the sub-papillary network lies close to the epithelium and provides a principal route for the supply of metabolites to that tissue. Capillary loops arising from this network run up into the connective tissue papillae; in the gingiva these sub-epithelial capillary loops are the largest in the body, originating at the junction of the attached and free gingiva and extending to the gingival crest. The tongue has a rich capillary system, extending into the lingual papillae, particularly the fungiform type.

Blood from the capillary beds is collected by a series of venules in the reticular layer of the lamina propria which connect with veins accompanying the arteries beneath the mucosa. Almost all the venous return is eventually carried by the internal jugular vein. Lymphatic capillaries are also present in the lamina propria and arise as blind beginnings in the papillae; these drain into larger vessels in the sub-mucosa. The superficial lymphatics accompany veins and the deep lymphatics accompany arteries except for the lymphatics draining the tongue which do not follow arteries or veins. All the lymphatic vessels ultimately drain into the deep cervical lymph nodes.

Anastomoses exist between small arteries and small veins and between metarterioles and venules; the latter connection provides a direct pathway, avoiding capillary beds, called a preferential channel or thoroughfare. In skin, where the blood flow plays an important role in controlling body temperature, there are highly specialized vessels, the arterio-venous shunts, that enable blood to by-pass capillary beds. Typical arterio-venous shunts have been described in the tongue of some mammals but not so far in the human oral mucosa so there is no reason to ascribe a role in thermo-regulation to the vascular system of this region.

4:5 Innervation of the oral mucosa

The oral mucosa, in keeping with its sensory function, has numerous sensory nerves together with some autonomic fibres (chiefly sympathetic) supplying smooth muscle and glands. Most of the sensory innervation is provided by the trigeminal nerve (5th cranial nerve) although afferent fibres also reach the brain via the 7th, 9th and 10th cranial nerves.

The sensory nerves form a network within the reticular layer of the lamina propria and a fine subepithelial plexus can also be seen. Thin unmyelinated nerves that are present in the adventitia of the blood vessels belong

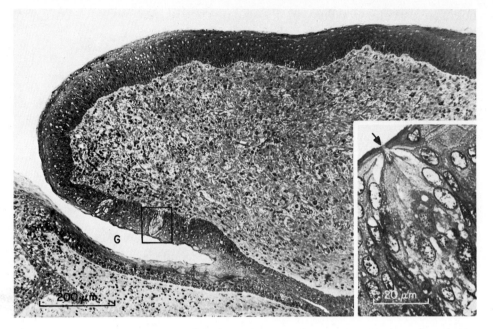

Fig. 24. A histological section showing taste buds present in the epithelium of a circumvallate papilla from the dorsum of the tongue (see also Fig. 27b). A deep groove (G) runs around the papilla into which empty the glands of von Ebner.

Inset: an enlarged view of a simple taste bud showing its barrel-like appearance and the apical pore (arrow).

to the autonomic nervous system. The nerve networks tend to be more concentrated and the sensory endings more numerous in the mucosa lining the anterior part of the oral cavity. This is particularly true at the tip of the tongue and on the rugal crest of the hard palate and corresponds with the greater tactile and thermal sensitivity of these regions.

Sensory nerves terminate in both free and organized endings. Free endings are simple non-myelinated terminations of the nerve fibres found in both the connective tissue and the epithelium (see Fig. 21)—some intra-epithelial nerve endings seem to be associated with Merkel cells (see Chapter 3, section 4). Organized nerve endings are more complex; they are only found in the lamina propria, usually in the papillary region, and consist of a coiled fibre or group of fibres that may be enclosed in a connective tissue capsule. Various types of ending each having a characteristic morphology have been described; these include the Meissner and Ruffini corpuscles, Krause end-bulbs and muco-cutaneous end organs. However it is now generally accepted that a particular type of ending is not exclusively associated with a particular sensory modality so that less reliance is placed on an elaborate morphological classification of sensory endings. As all the endings described above are terminal portions of the afferent fibres they can both detect and transmit stimuli directly. While the different sensory modalities do not have specific receptors they probably have specific fibres.

The lips, anterior palate and tip of the tongue are most sensitive to touch, having a greater sensitivity than the fingertips. Touch receptors in the soft palate and in the oropharynx initiate swallowing, gagging and retching reflexes. Temperature receptors, which are of two kinds, one sensitive to warmth and the other to cold, are most numerous in the anterior parts of the tongue and oral mucosa; these regions are the most sensitive, the lips being comparable in sensitivity to the eyelids. Pain is detected by the free endings of specific fibres but little is known about their distribution in the oral cavity, although some areas, such as the gingivae, seem to be particularly insensitive. However, painful stimuli do lead to jaw opening and salivation reflexes.

There are two specialized types of *sensory cell* also found in oral mucosa; the Merkel cell which is concerned with sensitivity to touch, and the taste bud. Both these cells receive stimuli which are subsequently relayed to the afferent neurone.

Taste buds are found in the mucosa of the tongue, soft palate and pharynx, the majority being present within the epithelium of the lingual papillae (Fig. 24). Taste buds are characteristically barrel shaped structures, consisting of 30–60 spindle shaped cells tapering towards the apex of the bud where they converge to form a pore (inset, Fig. 24). These cells have been described as 'light' or 'dark' according to their histological staining but the functional significance of the two types of cell is unclear. Although nerve fibres are associated with these cells it is not known whether the fibres themselves are directly stimulated by taste or whether the cells act as sensory receptors. The basic modalities of taste, salty, sweet, sour and bitter, may each be detected by different lingual papillae, and taste buds in different regions of the oral cavity may have different sensitivities to a given modality. Taste buds on the tongue seem more sensitive to salty and sweet modalities, those on the palate to sour and bitter. There are also receptors that respond to water taste and play a role in signalling the assuagance of thirst; these occur in the larynx or circumvallate papillae of some animals but their location in the oral cavity of man is uncertain.

Further reading

BARRETT A.J. (1971) The biochemistry and function of mucosubstances. *Histochem. J.* **3**, 213–221.

FARBMAN A.I. & ALLGOOD J.P. (1971) Innervation, sensory receptors and sensitivity of the oral mucosa. In *Current Concepts of the Histology of Oral Mucosa* (edited by Squier, C.A. and Meyer, J.) 250–273, Thomas, Springfield, Ill.

FULMER H.M., SHEETZ T.H. & NARKATES A.J. (1974) Oxytalan connective tissue fibres: a review. *J. Oral Path.* **3**, 291–316.

MELCHER A.H. & EASTOE J.E. (1969) Connective tissue of the periodontium. In *Biology of the Periodontium* (edited by Melcher, A.H. and Bowen, W.H.) 167–344, Academic Press, London.

WEISS L. (1972) *The cells and tissues of the immune system.* Prentice Hall, New Jersey.

CHAPTER 5
THE INTERFACE BETWEEN EPITHELIUM AND CONNECTIVE TISSUE

The region where the oral epithelium meets the connective tissue is an irregular interface at which the upward projections of the connective tissue papillae interdigitate with the downward projecting epithelial ridges. The frequency, extent and shape of the interdigitations vary in different regions of the oral mucosa but in all areas provide a greater area of interface between the epithelium and connective tissue than is present between the surface of the epithelium and the exterior. This configuration therefore plays an important role in distributing mechanical stress applied to the surface of the epithelium over a wide area of the supporting tissues and, since the surface layers of the epithelium are relatively impermeable, in providing the major route for metabolic exchange with the epithelium. Thus the interface serves both metabolic and mechanical functions.

There are differences between the configuration of the connective tissue-epithelium interface in masticatory and in lining mucosa which may reflect different mechanical properties; in the masticatory mucosa the ridges are numerous, tall and narrow, while in lining mucosa they are less numerous, broader and shorter. As a consequence, the area of interface between the epithelium and connective tissue per unit of epithelial surface is much greater in masticatory mucosa than in lining mucosa and so provides for a stronger junctional attachment.

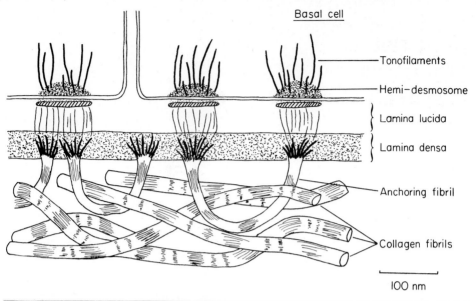

Basal cell

Tonofilaments

Hemi-desmosome

} Lamina lucida

} Lamina densa

Anchoring fibril

Collagen fibrils

100 nm

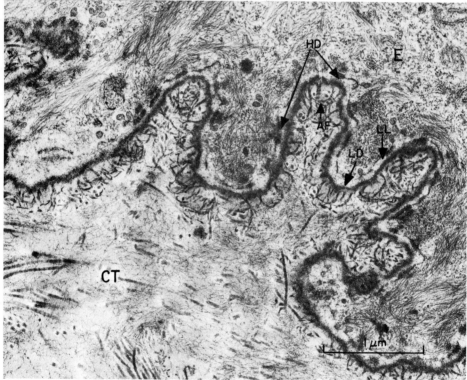

Fig. 25. The basal complex. The diagram depicts the organization of the junction between the epithelium and connective tissue. Below, on a slightly reduced scale, is an electron micrograph of this region in buccal epithelium: E = epithelium; CT = connective tissue; HD = hemi-desmosomes; LD = lamina densa; LL = lamina lucida; AF = anchoring fibrils.

5:1 The basement membrane

The term basement membrane has been used at a histological level to describe the junction between epithelium and connective tissue that appears as a continuous but relatively structureless layer some 1–2 µm thick after treatment with periodic-acid Schiff (paS) or silver stains.

Ultrastructural examination of the basement membrane in a number of tissues, including oral mucosa, has revealed an essentially similar organization in each case which is illustrated in Fig. 25. Running parallel with the basal plasma membranes of the basal epithelial cells and separated from them by a relatively clear zone some 20–80 nm wide is a dense layer, 20–70 nm thick; these two layers have been called the *lamina lucida* and *lamina densa* respectively. Associated with the lamina densa are striated fibrils, called *anchoring fibrils*, which loop beneath the lamina densa and through which run some of the collagen fibrils of the connective tissue. Where the end of each anchoring fibril enters the lamina densa it fans out to form a spray of finer filaments which, it has been suggested, traverse the lamina lucida and terminate opposite the intercellular plaques of the hemidesmosomes of the basal cells.

From the above account it is apparent that the basement membrane is not a membrane at all in ultrastructural terms but a complex of fibrils which interlock collagen fibrils of the connective tissue with the lamina densa and lamina lucida, and possibly with the epithelium. It is thus more appropriate to use the terms *basal lamina* or *basal complex* when referring to the structure observed in the electron microscope. The basement membrane seen in the light microscope is obviously a very much larger structure than the basal complex described by electron microscopists, and it would seem that the histological staining reactions used to demonstrate the basement membrane also stain the anchoring fibrils and some of the associated sub-epithelial collagen fibrils, which are often classified as 'reticulin fibres' (see Chapter 4, section 2).

Chemically, the basal complex consists predominantly of protein fibrils in a glycoprotein matrix. Although it was originally thought to be a condensation of polymerized connective tissue ground substance and fibrils, there is now considerable evidence that the lamina densa is a secretory product of the epithelial cells, as similar structures are formed by epithelia lacking any contact with connective tissue, such as at the enamel surface of the tooth (see Chapter 6, section 4). However the anchoring fibrils are probably products of the connective tissue so the whole basal complex represents a combined product of the epithelium and connective tissue.

5:2 Functions of the basal complex

Although a complete basal complex is not developed in embryonic oral mucosa until after the entry of immigrant cells such as the melanocyte and Langerhans cell, it seems certain that the structure is not able to limit the subsequent movement of cells into the epithelium. Inflammatory cells are not an unusual sight in the epithelium and their entry is associated with breaks in the basal complex. However at the molecular level it is likely that a continuous basal lamina can exert a filtering effect, and supplement the barrier function of the superficial layers of the epithelium.

The basal complex also has a role to play in attaching the epithelium to the connective tissue. Two factors appear to be largely responsible for this union, one being the adhesion between the epithelial cells and the lamina densa and the other the attachment of the lamina densa to the subjacent connective tissue. The material constituting the lamina densa has many similarities to the intercellular cement substance found between epithelial cells, so that adhesion may occur between the basal cells and the lamina densa as it does between the epithelial cells. The lamina densa in turn is attached to the underlying collagen of the connective tissue by the system of anchoring fibrils. When oral epithelium is separated experimentally from its connective tissue by means of suction applied to the epithelial surface, the epithelial cells at first only remain attached at the sites of the hemi-desmosomes. Eventually a blister is created by the complete separation of the epithelium at the level of the lamina lucida, the lamina densa usually remaining attached to the connective tissue by the anchoring fibrils. In the blisters that are typically formed in the disease pemphigoid, there is a separation of the epithelium from the connective tissue at the level of the basal complex although the reason for the separation is uncertain; some evidence suggests that anti-basement membrane antibodies are present in affected persons and the destruction of the region has an immunological basis.

Further reading

FRITHIOF L. (1969) Ultrastructure of the basement membrane in normal and hyperplastic human oral epithelium compared with that in pre-invasive and invasive carcinoma. *Acta. Path. Microbiol. Scand. Suppl.* **200.**

SUSI F.R. (1971) The basal lamina and its fibrils. In *Current Concepts of the Histology of Oral Mucosa* (edited by Squier, C.A. and Meyer, J.) 173–180. Thomas, Springfield, Ill.

CHAPTER 6
REGIONAL DIFFERENCES OF THE ORAL MUCOSA

The range of regional variation seen in oral mucosa is, if we exclude appendages such as nails and hair, even greater than that seen in the skin. This range includes differences not only in the composition of the lamina propria and the form of the epithelial-connective tissue junction but also in the type of covering epithelium, which can show a wide variation in thickness and in the prevalence and type of keratinization. There are also differences in the nature of the sub-mucosa and the way in which the mucosa is attached to underlying structures. It is commonplace to regard these regional differences as representing functional adaptations and to classify oral mucosa into three functional types, *masticatory mucosa*, *lining mucosa* and *specialized mucosa*; the main features of each type are summarized in Table 4 and the regions of the oral cavity occupied by each type of mucosa have already been illustrated diagrammatically in Fig. 1. Furthermore, there are several regions of particular morphological and clinical significance which will be described separately.

6:1 Masticatory mucosa

Masticatory mucosa is present in those areas of the oral cavity exposed to the compression and shear forces of mastication, such as the hard palate and gingiva. While the dorsum of the tongue might also be included in this

Table 4. Structure of mucosa within different regions of the oral cavity.

Region	Mucosa			
	Covering epithelium	Lamina propria		Sub-mucosa

Region	Covering epithelium	Lamina propria	Sub-mucosa
1. Lining mucosa			
Soft palate	Thin (approx. 150 µm) non-keratinized stratified squamous; taste buds present	Thick with numerous short papillae; elastic fibres forming an elastic lamina; highly vascular with well developed capillary network	Diffuse tissue containing numerous minor salivary glands (mucous)
Ventral surface of tongue	Thin non-keratinized stratified squamous	Thin with numerous short papillae and some elastic fibres; a few minor salivary glands (mucous, serous and mixed); capillary network in subpapillary layer, reticular layer relatively avascular	No distinct layer—the mucosa is bound to the connective tissue surrounding the tongue musculature
Floor of mouth	Very thin (approx. 100 µm) non-keratinized stratified squamous	Short broad papillae; some elastic fibres; extensive vascular supply with short, anastomosing capillary loops	Loose fibrous connective tissue containing fat, the sub-lingual and minor salivary glands (predominantly mucous)
Alveolar mucosa	Thin non-keratinized stratified squamous	Papillae are short or absent; connective tissue containing many elastic fibres; capillary loops close to the surface supplied by vessels running superficially to the periosteum	Loose connective tissue, containing thick elastic fibres, attaching it to periosteum of alveolar process; minor salivary glands (mixed)
Labial and buccal mucosa	Very thick (approx. 500 µm) non-keratinized stratified squamous (often para-keratinized in occlusal plane)	Short, irregular papillae; dense fibrous connective tissue containing collagen and some elastic fibres; rich vascular supply giving off anastomosing capillary loops into papillae	Mucosa firmly attached to underlying muscle by collagen and elastin; dense collagenous connective tissue with fat, minor salivary glands, sometimes sebaceous glands
Lips; vermilion border	Thin ortho-keratinized stratified squamous	Long narrow papillae; capillary loops in papillary layer close to surface	Mucosa firmly attached to underlying muscle; some sebaceous glands on vermilion border, minor salivary glands and fat in intermediate zone
intermediate zone	Thin para-keratinized stratified squamous	Long irregular papillae; elastic and collagen fibres in connective tissues	

Table 4. Continued.

Region	Mucosa		Sub-mucosa
	Covering epithelium	Lamina propria	
2. Masticatory mucosa			
Gingiva	Thick (approx. 250 μm), ortho-keratinized and para-keratinized stratified squamous, often showing a stippled surface	Long narrow papillae; dense collagenous connective tissue; not highly vascular but long capillary loops with numerous anastomoses particularly on crevicular aspect	Mucosa firmly attached by collagen fibres to cementum and periosteum of alveolar process ('mucoperiosteum'); no glands, fat or muscle
Hard palate	Thick, ortho-keratinized stratified squamous thrown into transverse palatine ridges (rugae)	Long papillae; thick dense collagenous tissue, especially under rugae; moderate vascular supply with short capillary loops	Dense collagenous connective tissue attaching mucosa to periosteum ('mucoperiosteum'); anteriorly fat, posteriorly minor salivary glands are packed into the connective tissue
3. Specialized mucosa			
Dorsal surface of tongue	Thick, keratinized stratified squamous forming three types of lingual papillae some bearing taste buds	Long papillae; mucous and serous glands (von Ebners glands); lymphoid tissue (lingual tonsils) posteriorly; rich innervation especially near taste buds; capillary plexus in papillary layer, large vessels lying deeper	No distinct layer, the mucosa is bound to the connective tissue surrounding the musculature of the tongue

category because of its role in mastication, it has a rather specialized structure and is considered separately. Masticatory mucosa lines immobile structures such as the palate and alveolar processes and is firmly bound to them, either by a fibrous sub-mucosa or directly, by attachment of the lamina propria to the periosteum of underlying bone, as in the gingiva and parts of the hard palate. This latter arrangement is termed a muco-periosteum (see Fig. 4(c)). The lamina propria is thick, containing a dense network of collagen fibres in the form of large closely packed bundles. These follow a direct course between their anchoring points so that there is relatively little slack to be taken up and the tissue does not yield on impact—this enables the mucosa to resist heavy loading. The junction with the overlying epithelium shows a highly convoluted interface because of the many deep rete pegs which may serve to increase the area available for mechanical attachment of the epithelium and so help resist its stripping off under shear forces.

The epithelial surface of masticatory mucosa is ortho-keratinized in the hard palate and over most of the gingiva although large areas of the gingiva are para-keratinized in many individuals. These surfaces are stiff and inextensible and well suited to withstand abrasion by food particles during mastication.

An extreme example of masticatory mucosa is found in areas of the hard palate where an ortho-keratinized epithelium covers a dense, fibrous connective tissue. This in turn overlays areas of fat or glandular tissue in the sub-mucosa which act as a cushion, so that the mucosa can bear the mechanical loads imposed upon it, as happens when food is being pressed between the dorsum of the tongue and the palate during mastication, without being unduly compressed against the underlying bone.

6:2 Lining mucosa

Some areas of the oral mucosa such as those covering the lips, cheeks, underside of tongue, floor of mouth and the alveolar processes as far as the gingiva, are highly mobile and undergo considerable distension as the result of muscular movement. These regions together with the soft palate are designated as lining mucosa. In

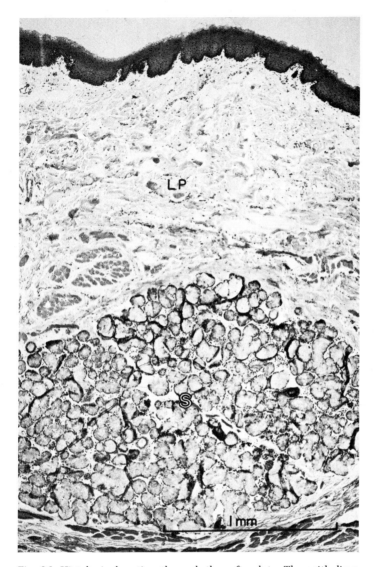

Fig. 26. Histological section through the soft palate. The epithelium is non-keratinized with short blunt ridges and there is a thick lamina propria (LP). A minor salivary gland (S) is present beneath the mucosa.

all these regions the epithelium is non-keratinized but thicker than in masticatory mucosa, sometimes exceeding 500 μm in the cheek. This type of surface is pliable and adapted for elongation. The junction with the connective tissue is relatively smooth showing few rete pegs, which are short and wide.

The lamina propria consists of a much thicker layer than in masticatory mucosa and contains fewer collagen fibres which follow a more irregular course between anchoring points. This allows for considerable distension of the mucosa before they become taut and so limit further extension. Associated with the collagen are numerous elastic fibres (which are comparatively sparse in masticatory mucosa) which tend to control the deformation of the mucosa as it is stretched until the collagen fibres become taut and limit further extension. Where the mucosa covers muscle, it is tightly attached by a mixture of collagen and elastic fibres; these latter fibres retract the mucosa towards the muscle as it becomes slack, and so prevent it bulging outwards between the teeth and being bitten. Thus in the lips and cheeks the mucosa follows the movements of the musculature very closely and they function as combined structures. The mucosa of the underside of the tongue, although having a thin epithelium and lamina propria is also tightly bound to the underlying muscle. On the other hand the alveolar mucosa and that covering the floor of the mouth are very loosely attached to the underlying structures via a thick sub-mucosa; in this case it is the elastic fibres present in the lamina propria that tend to restore the mucosa to its resting position after distension. Intermediate between the above types of lining mucosa is the mucosa of the soft palate (Fig. 26) which is flexible but not highly mobile and separated from the loose and highly glandular sub-mucosa by a layer of elastic fibres.

6:3 Specialized mucosa*

There are some areas of oral mucosa which show such specialized organization that their classification as either lining or masticatory mucosa is inappropriate.

The mucosa covering the dorsal surface of the tongue is unlike that anywhere else in the oral cavity in that it has different kinds of lingual papillae, some of which have a mechanical function, while others bear taste buds that have a sensory function (Fig. 27).

The anterior and posterior parts of the tongue have different embryological origins, and the posterior third, extending backwards from the V-shaped groove of the

*This section contributed by Nicola M. Grover-Johnson, Dept. Neuropathology, New York University Medical Center, New York.

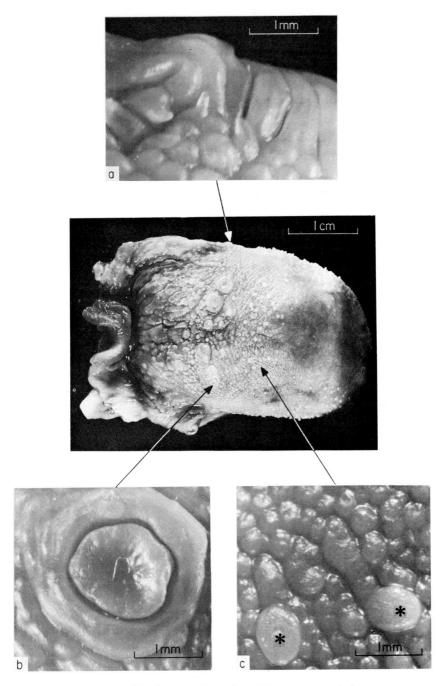

Fig. 27. A photograph of the dorsal surface of a child's tongue (centre) showing the distribution and types of lingual papillae. The ridge shaped foliate papillae are located laterally (a) while circumvallate papillae (b) are situated in a row in front of the sulcus terminalis. Fungiform papillae are interspersed among the numerous filiform papillae on the anterior of the tongue, two of which are shown (asterisks) in (c).

sulcus terminalis contains a large amount of lymphoid tissue. In and around the sulcus terminalis are 8–12 large *circumvallate papillae* (Fig. 27), each surrounded by a deep circular groove into which open the ducts of the serous glands of von Ebner. These papillae have a connective tissue core which is covered with keratinized epithelium on the superior surface. The epithelium of the lateral walls of the papillae is non-keratinized and taste buds are present (see Fig. 24). *Foliate papillae* (Fig. 27a) occur laterally on the posterior part of the tongue although they are not invariably present. They consist of 4–11 parallel ridges that bound deep folds of the mucosa. The few taste buds present are found in the epithelium of the lateral walls of the ridges.

At the tip of the tongue, scattered singly between the filiform papillae are the smooth, *red fungiform papillae* (Fig. 27c). Their red coloration is due to the highly vascular connective tissue core showing through a thin non-keratinized covering epithelium. Taste buds are normally present in the epithelium on the superior surface of these papillae. *Filiform papillae* cover the anterior part of the tongue and consist of pointed cone-shaped papillae containing a core of connective tissue over which is a keratinized epithelium. They provide a tough abrasive surface that can be used to compress and break food when the tongue is apposed to the palatal surface. Although covered dorsally by what, functionally, is masticatory mucosa, the tongue is highly extensible and it is regions of non-specialized mucosa between the papillae that accommodate the marked changes in shape of the tongue.

6:4 Junctions of particular significance

In several regions of the oral cavity there are abrupt junctions between different tissues that are of both morphological interest and of practical importance to the clinician.

6:4:1 THE MUCO-CUTANEOUS JUNCTION

At the lips the skin, containing hairs, sebaceous glands and sweat glands, passes into a transitional zone in which hairs and sweat glands are lacking although occasional sebaceous glands are present, particularly at

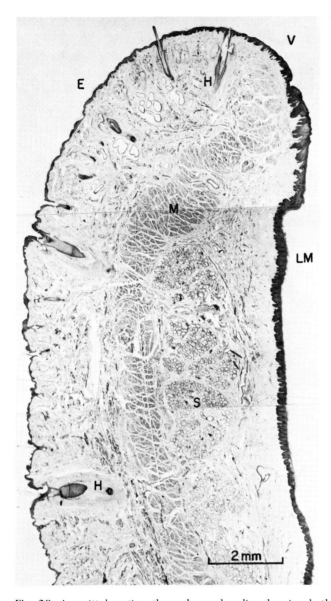

Fig. 28. A sagittal section through monkey lip, showing both skin and oral mucosa between which lies the vermilion border (V). The epidermis (E) is much thinner than the epithelium of the labial mucosa (LM) and contains several hair follicles (H). Several groups of minor salivary glands (S) are present beneath the oral mucosa as well as portions of the orbicularis oris muscle (M).

the angle of the mouth (Fig. 28). The epithelium of this region is thin but keratinized and there are long connective tissue papillae in which capillary loops run close to the epithelium. This vascular pattern, with the thin overlying epithelium, is responsible for the strong red coloration of the area which is often called the red zone, or *vermilion border*, of the lip. Between the vermilion border and the thicker non-keratinized oral labial mucosa is an intermediate zone which in adults is covered by a para-keratinized epithelium. In infants this region is thickened as an adaptation to suckling.

6:4:2 THE MUCO-GINGIVAL JUNCTION

Although there are several sites where masticatory mucosa meets lining mucosa, that where the attached gingiva meets the alveolar mucosa is the most abrupt. Clinically, the junction is marked by a slight indentation,

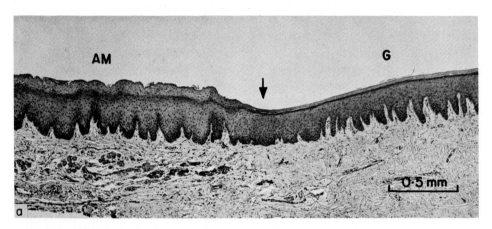

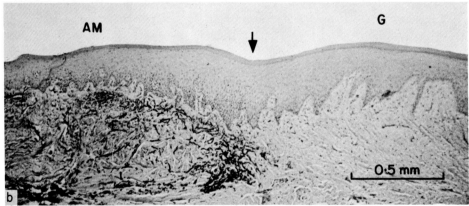

Fig. 29. The muco-gingival junction. The micrograph in (a) shows the abrupt transition (arrow) between the keratinized gingiva (G) on the right and the thicker non-keratinized alveolar mucosa (AM) on the left. Elastic fibres (E) are abundant in the alveolar mucosa but not the gingiva as can be seen in (b) where the tissue has been stained with Hart's elastin stain.

the *muco-gingival groove*, and by a change in colour from the bright pink of the highly vascular alveolar mucosa to the paler, less vascular, attached gingiva (see Fig. 2). At this junction not only is there a change in the type of epithelium from keratinized to a thicker non-keratinized type but also a marked contrast in the composition of the connective tissue (Fig. 29a). The lamina propria of attached gingiva contains numerous coarse bundles of collagen fibres and is firmly bound to the periosteum of the alveolar bone to form a muco-periosteum; the lamina propria of alveolar mucosa has numerous elastic fibres which also extend into the thick sub-mucosal region. This contrast is seen very clearly in sections through the junction stained to show elastic fibres (Fig. 29b). As the alveolar mucosa is not directly attached to muscle, these elastic fibres serve to restore it to its original state after distension by the action of muscles in and around the lips.

6:4:3 THE DENTO-GINGIVAL JUNCTION

The region where the oral mucosa meets the surface of the tooth (Fig. 30) is of considerable importance as it is a potentially weak spot in the otherwise continuous epithelial lining of the oral cavity. While it is clear that many of the collagen fibres of the lamina propria of free gingiva insert directly into the cementum of the tooth, controversy has existed for decades as to whether there is structural organic union between the oral epithelium and the dental hard tissue or whether it is merely held in close apposition to the tooth by pressures within the connective tissue. As it is this junction between the epithelium and the enamel that is the principal seal between the oral cavity and the underlying tissues, it is important to have an understanding of the nature of this union, and recent ultrastructural studies have now substantially resolved the issue.

In the average human mouth, in which mild gingival inflammation is invariably present, the gingival sulcus is of the order of 0·1–1·0 mm in depth; where complete absence of inflammation is achieved the sulcus may virtually disappear. The floor of the sulcus and the epithelium cervical to it, which is applied to the tooth surface, has in the past been called the 'epithelial attachment'. It is now termed *junctional epithelium*.

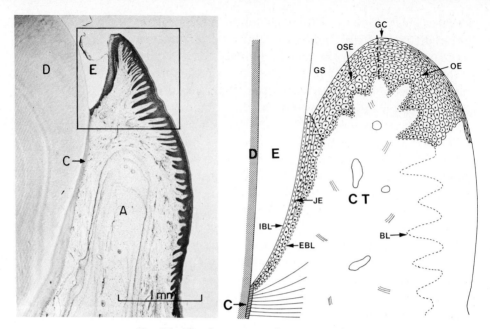

Fig. 30. The dento-gingival junction. The micrograph on the left shows a decalcified section through the tooth and its supporting tissues (A = alveolar bone; C = cementum; D = dentine; E = enamel).

The area in the square is depicted in the diagram on the right, which shows in particular the different types of epithelium: oral epithelium (OE); oral sulcular epithelium (OSE) and junctional epithelium (JE). The junctional epithelium is attached to the enamel via the internal basal lamina (IBL) and to the connective tissue via the external basal lamina (EBL) which is continuous with the basal lamina (BL) of the rest of the epithelium. (CT = connective tissue; GC = gingival crest; GS = gingival sulcus.) The diagram is reproduced with permission from the *British Medical Bulletin*, **31**, 169 (1975).

The walls of the sulcus are lined by epithelium derived from, and continuous with, that of the rest of the oral mucosa. This has been designated *oral sulcular epithelium* and has the same basic structure as non-keratinized oral epithelium, the ortho- or para-keratinized surface of the free gingiva stopping at the level of the gingival crest.

Junctional epithelium is derived from the reduced enamel epithelium of the tooth germ. It consists of flattened cells aligned parallel to the tooth surface and tapering from 1–2 layers in thickness apically to 15–30 layers coronally. The epithelium has a smooth connective tissue interface where there is a normal basal lamina, designated the *external basal lamina*, with associated hemi-desmosomes. Between the plasma membrane of the junctional epithelial cells and the enamel

84

surface a similar *internal basal lamina* is present, situated on the actual enamel (or cementum) surface and again associated with hemi-desmosomes on the membranes of the epithelial cells. The union between the epithelium and tooth is thus mediated by structures similar to those that attach epithelium to connective tissue elsewhere in the oral mucosa.

The junctional epithelium is not simply an area of non-keratinized oral epithelium—it has particularly wide intercellular spaces and lacks the numbers of tonofilaments seen in cells in other regions of oral epithelium. Although its cells divide and migrate to the surface, they show no sign of differentiation to form a keratinized surface epithelium. These features, as well as the frequent presence of neutrophil leucocytes and mononuclear cells may all contribute to the apparent permeability of the tissue. This has been extensively studied and a variety of substances ranging from cells to tissue fluid and small protein molecules have been shown to be capable of traversing the epithelium (see Chapter 3, section 5). This makes the structure of the sulcus an important factor when considering the aetiology and pathogenesis of periodontal disease.

Further reading

BINNIE W.H. & LEHNER T. (1970) Histology of the muco-cutaneous junction at the corner of the human mouth. *Archs. oral Biol.* **15**, 777–786.

LOZDAN J. & SQUIER C.A. (1969) The histology of the muco-gingival junction. *J. Periodont. Res.* **4**, 83–93.

SCAPINO R.P. (1971) Biomechanics of masticatory and lining mucosa. In *Current Concepts of the Histology of Oral Mucosa* (edited by Squier, C.A. and Meyer, J.) 181–202. Thomas, Springfield, Ill.

SCHROEDER H.E. & LISTGARTEN M.A. (1971) *Fine Structure of the Developing Epithelial Attachment of Human Teeth*, Karger, Basel.

CHAPTER 7
METABOLISM OF THE ORAL
MUCOSA

7:1 Principal metabolic pathways in the oral mucosa

The tissues of the oral mucosa, like other tissues in the body, require a supply of metabolic substrates, inter-mediates and energy in order to maintain their structural integrity. In particular, oral epithelium, with a constantly renewing cell population which has a high rate of turnover, might be expected to be metabolically more active than its supporting connective tissues with a somewhat low rate of cell turnover. In addition to cell division there are in the epithelium the metabolic events accompanying differentiation which involve both synthesis and degradation, while in the connective tissues, fibres and ground substance are constantly turning over. The metabolism of oral mucosa reflects all these activities.

Studies on the metabolism of skin and oral mucosa supplement histological findings and provide information on the mechanisms involved in maintaining normal structure and function as well as aiding interpretation of the clinical and histological changes manifest as a result of, for example, altered endocrine or nutritional status, ageing and disease. However, much of the research on oral mucosa has been limited to the study of carbohydrate metabolism, seeking to compare activities of oral epithelium and connective tissue, of keratinized and non-keratinized regions and of the different cell layers of the epithelium.

Experimental approaches to this problem have been two-fold; attempts to measure the levels of activity of

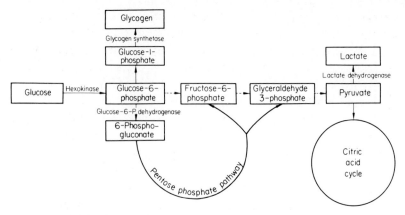

Fig. 31. The main routes for the metabolism of glucose.

various enzymes in the tissues—both by histochemistry and more recently by microchemistry (a combination of micro-dissection and ultramicrochemical assay—see Appendix 1) and assessments of the rate of metabolism of the tissue by measuring the uptake of a substrate or the accumulation of products of a metabolic pathway.

In order to illustrate these approaches it is perhaps useful to first remind the reader of the main pathways that glucose can follow on entering a cell. These are summarized in Fig. 31. The principal pathway is *glycolysis* (Embden-Meyerhof pathway) which under anaerobic conditions leads to the accumulation of lactic acid. Under aerobic conditions, lactate is not formed but pyruvate from glycolysis is further oxidized by the *citric acid cycle* (Krebs cycle; tricarboxylic acid cycle) which is the main energy-producing pathway of many cells. Under certain conditions, glucose-6-phosphate may by-pass the first steps of glycolysis and enter the *pentose phosphate pathway* (hexose monophosphate shunt). This pathway provides the cell with $NADPH_2$ (a coenzyme needed for the synthesis of fatty acids) and also with a means of producing pentose sugars for nucleic acid synthesis. These are all catabolic pathways; glucose may also enter synthetic (or anabolic) pathways including *glycogenesis* (glycogen synthesis) as also shown in Fig. 31. Sugars for the synthesis of mucosubstances are provided by the pentose phosphate pathway and by glycolysis.

Amongst the first studies on oral mucosa were those which measured the rate of oxygen consumption using standard manometric techniques. Although the oxygen uptake was found to be considerably greater than that for skin, the rates were far lower than those of certain other tissues, such as the kidney or submaxillary gland. Oxygen uptake by the oral epithelium was found to be approximately three times that of its connective tissue element. Oxidative metabolic pathways are however likely to be of lesser importance than non-oxidative pathways in epithelial tissues where the majority of the cells have no direct access to the blood supply. Thus utilization of glucose might be expected to give a better indication of metabolic activity in this type of tissue. Studies on skin using radioactively labelled glucose indicate that over 70% of the glucose metabolized by epidermis may be converted to lactic acid, i.e. the main energy producing pathway is anaerobic glycolysis. Comparable data for oral mucosa are not available, although studies on rat palate showed the rate of glycolysis (approximately $0 \cdot 1 - 0 \cdot 2$ μmoles glucose/mg tissue/hr at $37°C$) to be comparable to that obtained for mouse ear under the same conditions. Whilst this type of approach is useful for determining the rate of metabolism in relatively large samples such as whole mucosa, it is less easy to apply to particular areas of tissue, e.g. the connective tissue of oral mucosa or isolated layers of the epithelium, as chemical separation or dissection techniques are likely to damage the tissue and cause loss of enzyme activity.

The techniques of quantitative histochemistry and microchemistry provide information on the localization of enzyme activity because they are performed on tissue sections or micro-dissected fragments of tissue. The results must nevertheless be interpreted with caution as such techniques can only measure the **potential** activity of the tissue i.e. whether or not a tissue possesses the enzymes to catalyse a particular series of reactions. The levels of enzyme measured *in vitro* do not necessarily reflect their activity in the intact living tissue where subtle control mechanisms, based upon the levels of substrate and product present in the cell, may be operating. These controls are mediated via certain 'key' or 'rate-limiting' enzymes present in each pathway.

The enzymes in oral mucosa that have been most studied are those most amenable to biochemical investigation and not necessarily the most significant. They fall into two groups, namely the lysosomal hydrolytic enzymes and the enzymes of intermediary carbohydrate

89

metabolism. The former group include acid phosphatase, non-specific esterase, aryl-sulphatase and β-glucuronidase, whilst those related specifically to carbohydrate metabolism include hexokinase*, aldolase, glyceraldehyde-3-phosphate dehydrogenase and lactate dehydrogenase from the glycolytic pathway, isocitrate dehydrogenase* and malate dehydrogenase from the citric acid cycle and glucose-6-phosphate dehydrogenase* and 6-phosphogluconate dehydrogenase* from the pentose phosphate pathway. However only those marked with an asterisk are 'rate-limiting' enzymes and therefore the most likely to reflect inherent differences in activity of the pathways.

With these limitations in mind we shall examine some of the findings. The activity of hydrolytic enzymes is almost entirely confined to lysosomes in the basal and prickle cells of the epithelium. In the granular layer of keratinized epithelium they are not exclusively associated with lysosomes and may be associated with the removal of organelles that takes place at this level. Hydrolytic enzymes are present in lysosomes in the cells of the connective tissue, particularly in macrophages and polymorphonuclear leucocytes.

Studies on the enzymes of glycolysis, the pentose phosphate pathway and the citric acid cycle indicate that the oral mucosa is equipped with the enzymes to carry out all these processes. Table 5 lists the activities of some of the enzymes of glucose metabolism that have been measured in rat keratinized gingival tissue. It can be seen that enzymes involved in *gluconeogenesis* (the production of glucose from pyruvate) are either absent or present in extremely low quantities as might be expected in this tissue. However, the levels of activity of different enzymes in the same pathway vary enormously, reinforcing the view that the activity of a pathway cannot be predicted from the absolute activity of individual enzymes in that pathway. In this tissue, as in others, the activity of regulatory enzymes is generally lower than that of non-regulatory enzymes. Nevertheless, the levels of enzymes of glucose metabolism in oral epithelial tissues tend to be higher than in their associated connective tissues when expressed per unit dry weight of tissue. Likewise it has been shown that, in general, enzyme activities found in oral epithelium exceed those found in the epidermis.

90

Table 5. Activities of some enzymes of glucose metabolism in rat gingiva (Data based on Simpson, J.W. (1974) *J. Dent. Res. 53*, 938).

ENZYME	PATHWAY	ACTIVITY (μ moles of product/min/gm wet weight tissue at 25°C)
Hexokinase*	Glycolysis	2·2
Glucosephosphate isomerase	Glycolysis	20·2
Phosphofructokinase*	Glycolysis	4·2
Aldolase	Glycolysis	1·8
Triosephosphate isomerase	Glycolysis	12·8
Phosphoglycerate kinase	Glycolysis	3·5
Phosphoglyceromutase	Glycolysis	2·0
Enolase	Glycolysis	5·8
Pyruvate kinase*	Glycolysis	4·5
Lactate dehydrogenase	Glycolysis	11·9
Fructose 1,6-diphosphatase*	Gluconeogenesis	not detected
Glucose-6-phosphatase*	Gluconeogenesis	not detected
Glucose-6-phosphate dehydrogenase*	Pentose phosphate pathway	2·05
6-Phosphogluconate dehydrogenase*	Pentose phosphate pathway	0·55
Pyruvate oxidase complex	Glycolysis→citric acid cycle	0·40

*Key or rate-limiting enzymes

The interpretation of data relating to different degrees of keratinization of oral epithelium, which it might be hoped would shed some light on the mechanisms of keratinization, is rendered difficult by the limited range of keratinization found in most laboratory animals. It is not really permissible to compare data from different species but there are a few studies in which enzyme activities in epithelia from different regions of the same animal have been compared. Thus the keratinized area of rabbit buccal mucosa was found to contain approximately 2–3 times as much acid phosphatase and twice as much glucose-6-phosphate dehydrogenase as non-keratinized regions of the same tissue while epidermis showed even greater levels of these two enzymes; this might suggest an association between these two enzymes and the process of keratinization.

A further aspect of this difference between non-keratinized and keratinized tissues lies in the pattern of enzyme activities between layers of the epithelium. In non-keratinized rabbit buccal epithelium the activity of acid phosphatase, lactate dehydrogenase, malate dehydrogenase and glucose-6-phosphate dehydrogenase were all found to decrease progressively from the basal

91

layer to the surface. Similarly in the keratinized tissues studied, which include rat palate and cheek as well as human, dog and monkey gingiva, lactate dehydrogenase, aldolase and malate and succinate dehydrogenase, as well as NADP-dependant isocitrate dehydrogenase (involved in fat synthesis), all decreased in activity towards the surface. However glucose-6-phosphate dehydrogenase consistently increased from the basal to spinous layers but then decreased towards the surface. Acid phosphatases increased towards the surface, reaching a peak in the granular layer.

The decrease in activity in both types of epithelium of enzymes involved in glycolysis and the citric acid cycle suggests that less energy is produced by the cells as they differentiate and this may parallel the decrease in number of mitochondria seen ultrastructurally as the cells progress through the tissue. This reduction could be due to a lower energy requirement (the cells have ceased division) or because the cells are further removed from substrate and oxygen supply in the connective tissue. On the other hand, in keratinizing epithelium, cells in the more superficial layers synthesize keratohyalin and tonofilaments and it is possible that the rise in pentose phosphate pathway activity seen in this tissue is associated with the keratinization process. The increase in acid phosphatase activity supports the observation that organelles are degraded during keratinization.

These findings corroborate many of the histological changes observed during keratinization and throw some light on the biochemistry of this process although there is clearly a need for more work examining other pathways such as glycogen metabolism, and those involving lipid, protein and mucosubstance synthesis.

7:2 The effects of nutritional deficiencies on the oral mucosa

The metabolic pathways of the oral mucosa can only function normally if there is an adequate supply of essential nutrients in the diet, adequate digestion and absorption from the gut, and an adequate blood supply to carry them to the tissues. Deficiencies in the diet or defects in any of these processes, or in the output of hormones or other factors which regulate such metabolic activities, lead to functional disturbances which, if sufficiently severe, produce clinically manifest disease. Whilst it is not the purpose of this volume to discuss disease processes, a brief survey of the most important nutrients and hormones in relation to mucosal function is relevant at this stage and may provide a basis for understanding the mechanisms of many oral mucosal diseases.

7:2:1 DIRECT LOCAL EFFECTS

Before proceeding to discuss systemic metabolic functions it is important to realize that the nature of an individual's diet may have important direct effects on oral mucosa. The most obvious of these is the relation between diet, the accumulation of bacterial plaque and the severity of gingival inflammation : diets rich in sticky, readily fermentable carbohydrate, particularly sucrose, favour the development of plaque because many plaque organisms rapidly convert this to complex extracellular polymers of glucose which contributes to the cohesion of the plaque and to its adhesion to tooth and gingiva.

Elsewhere in the oral mucosa, toxic factors may be of importance. For example, it has been suggested that the high prevalence of the disease known as submucous fibrosis in Indians may be due to contact with chillies in the diet; the irritant effect of tobacco smoke, possibly combined with that of alcohol, has long been implicated in the development of hyperkeratotic lesions and of oral cancer.

7:2:2 EFFECTS OF GENERALIZED MALNUTRITION

In those communities where serious undernourishment is found, affected individuals show obvious changes such as wasting in adults and failure to thrive in children. The skin becomes thin and wrinkled, though oedema (famine oedema)—an accumulation of extracellular fluid due to disturbance in osmotic balance of the blood—may be present in many tissues. In such severe cases the nutritional deficiency is multiple—protein, calorie, vitamin and mineral—and the effects are non-specific with many metabolic activities disturbed. The oral mucosa shares in these effects which amount, in a word, to atrophy. Thus the epithelium will become thinner, due to a reduction in the size of individual cells and to a reduction in cell proliferation with fewer layers being present. Surface squames may accumulate leading to the appearance of scaling and flaking, and the mucosa is dry due to diminished activity of salivary glands. The corium will show decreased cellularity and vascularity and a relative increase in water content. This spectrum of atrophic change is present to some degree in the oral mucosa of aged individuals (see Chapter 8, section 3) and is mimicked by malabsorption syndromes due to diseases of the gastro-intestinal tract. Not surprisingly atrophic mucosa shows reduced resistance to injury and delayed healing.

Amino acids and proteins. In children suffering from the severe protein-calorie deficiency disease known as Kwashiorkor, seen in parts of Africa, normal commensal organisms of the mouth may invade the tissues producing extensive necrosis—a condition called cancrum oris.

Fatty acids. Whilst there is experimental evidence from animal studies to show that low fat diets and deprivation of essential fatty acids produces defects in oral tissues, the problem in Western countries now is more one of damage to health by excessive fat intake. Generalized obesity and accelerated development of arteriosclerosis is reflected in oral mucosa by increased deposits of adipose tissue in the sub-mucosa and thickening of the intima of arterioles.

7:2:3 VITAMINS

Vitamin A. Vitamin A has profound effects on the metabolism of epithelial tissues, deficiency resulting in hyperplasia and hyperkeratinization of many lining mucosae, and excess doses given to man and experimental animals, or applied to mucosa in organ cultures, resulting in thinning of the epithelium and a change in the differentiation of the epithelial cells from keratin-producing to mucus-secreting cells—this is called mucous metaplasia.

These effects have led to the implication of Vitamin A deficiency in the aetiology of hyperkeratotic lesions of the oral mucosa, and to the use of topical Vitamin A in their treatment, but the results are inconclusive. The vitamin may act by exerting a direct effect on the epithelial genome; lysosomal membranes also seem to be sensitive to altered levels of Vitamin A.

94

B-Group Vitamins. Vitamins of the B-complex, although different in chemical structure, have similar properties. Many are coenzymes of importance in intermediary metabolism.

Whilst certain specific diseases are recognized as due to deficiency of a particular B-group vitamin, for example beri-beri, due to thiamine deficiency, and pellagra, due to deficiency of nicotinic acid, in most cases in man the deficiency is multiple and may even involve protein-calorie deficiency as well. Specific oral manifestations of deficiency of thiamine, of riboflavin or of nicotinic acid have been described in experimental animals, and in man, but are not likely to be recognizable in clinical practice.

The clinical signs are those of atrophy and reduced resistance to infection and other local irritants. Thus the mucosa is thinner than normal with a reduced differentiation of epithelial cells—seen particularly in the tongue which loses its papillae and thus appears smooth. There is a widespread, diffuse, subepithelial inflammation (including glossitis, stomatitis and gingivitis) which possibly results from the penetration of irritants through an atrophic epithelium. Epithelial thinning and increased blood flow associated with the inflammation cause the tissues to appear much redder and the tissues are likely to be painful. Alterations in the balance of the oral microflora may result in superficial infections; for example angular cheilitis, associated with the fungus *Candida albicans.* Such patients may also show an increased susceptibility to develop acute necrotizing ulcerative gingivitis (Vincent's disease).

Folic acid deficiency in man produces a macrocytic anaemia, and deficiency of Vitamin B_{12} causes pernicious anaemia. Both may result in similar oral manifestations to deficiency of other B-group vitamins, exacerbated in this case by the local effect of the anaemia on the metabolism of oral mucosa. The tongue is characteristically affected, being red and sore in the early stages of the disease, and often patients complain of a burning sensation—glossodynia. In more advanced anaemia the atrophy is more marked and the tissues pale.

Vitamin C (ascorbic acid). Swelling and bleeding of the gingivae and loosening of the teeth are among the classical signs of the Vitamin C deficiency disease, scurvy. Ascorbic acid is essential for the oxidation of proline to hydroxyproline during the synthesis of collagen (see Chapter 4, section 2) so scurvy is a connective tissue disease, collagen synthesis being arrested at the proto-collagen stage, with the result that collagen is not available for growth, remodelling or repair following injury.

Severe deficiency of Vitamin C in both man and experimental animals has profound effects on oral tissues, particularly on the periodontium. There is reduced resistance to local irritants, for example dental plaque, and decreased capacity for repair. Whether or not minor deficiencies are of importance in oral disease in man is highly controversial. Extensive epidemiological investigations in several parts of the world have however failed to reveal an association between the severity of periodontal disease and levels of ascorbic acid in the body.

Vitamin D. In man this vitamin is largely synthesized in the skin, promoted by ultraviolet light, from sterol precursors derived from the diet; the oral mucosa presumably does not participate in this process. It is not known what role this vitamin plays in the maintenance of oral mucosa.

Vitamin E. Although deficiency of this vitamin in experimental animals results in sterility and muscular dystrophy and is thought by some to contribute to a 'youthful' appearance of skin, there is no satisfactory evidence for its being of importance in maintaining the functional integrity of skin and mucous membrane in man.

7:2:4 INORGANIC ELEMENTS

Of the many minerals and trace elements essential to life, two are of especial interest in relation to mucosal behaviour. These are iron and zinc.

Iron. Defects in the supply of iron to the body, or in its metabolism, result in iron-deficiency anaemia. The clinical oral manifestations are similar to those described above for other forms of anaemia and such patients are particularly prone to develop infective or other inflammatory lesions such as angular cheilitis and aphthous ulcers. It has been suggested that iron-deficiency anaemias predispose to the development of hyperkeratotic lesions in the mouth, some of which may eventually become malignant. Though the mechanism is not understood an association between iron-deficiency anaemia, glossitis, and dysphagia is well recognized—this is known as the Plummer-Vinson or Patterson-Kelly syndrome—and such patients are prone to develop carcinoma of the oesophagus.

Zinc. Although there is no information to suggest that the oral mucosa is involved in the zinc-deficiency syndromes that have been described in man, results from studies of zinc-deficient experimental animals have shown both an increase in cell proliferation in epidermis and oral epithelium and a conversion of ortho-keratinized epithelium to para-keratosis. These changes closely resemble the changes seen in psoriasis and certain keratotic lesions of the oral mucosa.

There is considerable evidence for the role of zinc preparations in promoting the healing of skin wounds and ulcers, and this beneficial effect has also been claimed for oral lesions. It is not clear how zinc participates in wound healing although it acts as a cofactor for a number of synthetic enzymes.

7:3 Hormonal influences on oral mucosa

Whilst the effects of some hormones are largely limited to specific target organs, many hormones have widespread effects on the metabolism of tissues throughout the body. Good examples of the former are the trophic hormones such as the adrenocorticotrophic hormone (ACTH) and thyrotrophin, and of the latter, thyroid hormone itself which influences the basal metabolic rate of the whole body, and insulin which controls carbohydrate utilization in many cells. Neither oral mucosa nor skin can be regarded as primary target organs for any hormone and the main effects of practical importance relate only to variations in the output of female sex hormones and of insulin, while the adrenal cortex and pituitary hormones have a marginal influence.

7:3:1 SEX HORMONES

Variations in the levels of the circulating sex hormones, androgens, oestrogens and progestogens, occur in both sexes at puberty and in females throughout the menstrual cycle, during pregnancy and at the menopause. Changes in the oral mucosa occur during all these phases.

Raised levels of oestrogens and progestogens influence nucleic acid synthesis. In oral epithelium this is reflected as increased mitotic activity resulting in hyperplasia and increased keratinization, and in the lamina propria as increased cellularity and synthetic activity. This latter process results in an increase in fibrous elements and in ground substance, particularly proteoglycans. Depressed levels have opposite effects.

Cyclical variations in the keratinization of oral mucosa have been reported to occur during the menstrual cycle. However, the influence of sex hormones is most clearly seen in post-menopausal women where atrophy of the oral mucosa is common and may be reversed to some extent by administration of oestrogens (see Chapter 8, section 3).

High levels of sex hormones increase the susceptibility of oral tissues to local irritants so that gingivitis, for example, is more severe at puberty, during pregnancy and in women taking oral contraceptive drugs. This is of great practical importance but it should be explained that the primary cause is the presence of bacterial plaque, so that inflammation can be readily controlled by good oral hygiene. Progestogenic hormones appear to exert the major influence, possibly by altering the structure and permeability of small blood vessels and by increasing the fragility of lysosomes in many connective tissue and inflammatory cells.

7:3:2 INSULIN

The importance of this hormone lies in the increased susceptibility to infection of diabetic subjects. The oral mucosa is no exception and periodontal disease and other lesions are more common; the initial lesion appears to be vascular with thickening of the walls of small blood vessels in gingiva and elsewhere. The disturbed water balance in this disease results in reduced salivary flow and dryness of the mouth.

7:3:3 ADRENAL CORTICOSTEROIDS

The widespread anti-anabolic and anti-inflammatory properties of corticosteroids are of no less importance in the oral mucosa than elsewhere. Where the balance of these hormones is altered the oral tissues may be more susceptible to disease, and healing may be impaired. Topical, and occasionally systemic, steroid therapy may be used in the treatment of those lesions of the oral mucosa with a suspected immune-inflammatory pathogenesis.

7:3:4 PITUITARY HORMONES

Of these, the melanocyte stimulating activity associated with the adrenocorticotrophic hormone is worthy of brief mention. In conditions where the output of the anterior pituitary is increased, usually due as in Addison's disease to chronic insufficiency of the adrenal cortex, then increased pigmentation may follow. The lips, cheeks and tongue are often affected; these are sites that are not often pigmented even in dark-skinned races.

Further reading

GERSON S. & MEYER I. (1970) Biochemical assay of heterogeneous soft tissues of the oral cavity. *Advances in Oral Biol.* **4**, 289–312.

JENKINS G.N. (1976) *The Physiology and Biochemistry of the Mouth.* 4th Edition. Blackwell Scientific Publications, Oxford.

WATERHOUSE J.P. (1969) Effect of endocrine secretions on the periodontium and its constituent tissues. In *Biology of The Periodontium* (edited by Melcher, A.H. and Bowen, W.H.) 453–483. Academic Press, London.

CHAPTER 8
DEVELOPMENT, EPITHELIAL-MESENCHYMAL INTERACTIONS AND AGE CHANGES IN ORAL MUCOSA*

We have already seen that, although all oral mucosa is composed of a stratified squamous epithelium on a similar connective tissue base, there are marked regional differences in structure, many of which are predetermined and develop early in intra-uterine life. Minor variations may be superimposed on this basic pattern— for example, in skin, callouses develop on hands and feet due to friction, and similarly, keratinization of the oral mucosa of the cheek may occur along the occlusal line.

The type of epithelium which develops in a particular site appears to be determined primarily by the connective tissue on which it rests—both during embryonic development and in the adult, and instructions pass between these two components of the mucous membrane throughout the life of the tissue. These so-called *epithelial-mesenchymal interactions* are considered in more detail later and we shall first describe briefly the developmental stages of oral mucosa.

8:1 Developmental stages of oral mucosa

The epithelium of most of the oral mucous membrane, like that of skin, is derived from embryonic ectoderm. Behind the primitive bucco-pharyngeal membrane it is derived from foregut endoderm and, although there is

*This chapter contributed by Margarete Hackemann, MRC Clinical Research Centre, Northwick Park, Middlesex.

some controversy as to the precise location of this membrane in man, structures derived from the internal surfaces of the branchial arches, such as the posterior portion of the tongue, floor of mouth and pharynx are lined by epithelium of endodermal origin. The connective tissue arises *in situ* from mesenchymal cells.

By the 3rd week of intra-uterine life the primitive oral cavity is lined by a simple ectodermal layer. Over the roof of the oral cavity this is a single layer of cuboidal cells and is continuous with a similar unicellular layer of embryonic ectoderm covering the external surface of the developing forebrain. Interestingly, in view of its ultimately greater thickness, the lateral borders of the oral cavity are already multi-layered, increasing from 2 cell layers at 3 weeks to 5 or more cell layers at 6 weeks.

At this early stage the future lamina propria is composed of a sub-ectodermal condensation of branching cells with a minimal, intercellular, fibrillar component. A more dense fibrillar accumulation along the epithelial interface heralds the development of the basement membrane.

At eight weeks *in utero* the palatal shelves close so that the future morphology of the oral cavity becomes recognizable. All areas are now lined by several layers of ectoderm and it becomes possible to distinguish sites destined for keratinization, such as the alveolar ridge and hard palate, from those which will remain non-keratinized, like cheek, lip and soft palate. In the former sites the basal cells are columnar, contain fine tonofilaments and have cytoplasmic processes which project into the mesenchyme.

At a similar stage, i.e. from eight weeks onwards, the skin surface has developed 3 layers; a basal germinative layer, an intermediate layer, and a surface layer known as *periderm*. The periderm is distinctive; it is composed of large bulbous cells, which give the surface an undulating appearance. Periderm cells are shed into the amniotic cavity throughout embryonic life and, although there is a progressive reduction in their size, the periderm remains as a distinctive structure until a keratinized layer has differentiated beneath it—usually by the 26th week—after which the periderm is shed.

Although the term periderm has also been used to describe the surface layer of developing oral epithelium

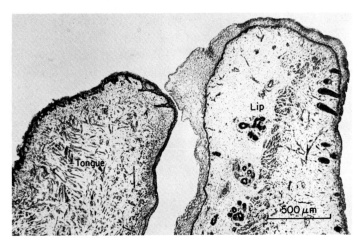

Fig. 32. A sagittal section through the lip and tongue of a human embryo of approximately 15 weeks. Differences are already apparent between areas destined to form a keratinized surface such as the dorsum of tongue and the epidermis of lip, and that forming the thicker, non-keratinized labial mucosa (compare with the fully developed lip in Fig. 28).

it is never as distinctive as it is on the embryonic skin surface. Between the 14th and 20th weeks (see Fig. 32) the oral epithelium increases in thickness up to 15 cell layers in places, the prickle cell character of the central cells becomes detectable, and desmosomes are well formed. In areas destined for keratinization the surface cells appear flattened and contain scattered kerato-hyalin granules. Toward the end of this period a distinct stratum granulosum can be seen and the surface layers are keratinized—though this is probably limited to para-keratosis and ortho-keratin is not thought to appear until 6 months after birth.

In the lamina propria, the network of widely spaced but interconnecting stellate cells begins to accumulate irregularly arranged intercellular fibres of reticulin between the 6th and 8th week. At this stage the primitive connective tissue of the lining mucosa of the lip and cheek is more loosely arranged and less cellular than that of the masticatory mucosa of the alveolar ridge and hard palate, in which collagen fibres can be detected from between the 8th and 11th week. In all regions small blood vessels are by now abundant.

By the 14th week most mesenchymal cells have lost contact with their neighbours and are recognizable as

103

fibroblasts. Collagen fibres increase in number and size, and a little later—between the 16th and 20th week—elastic fibres appear, but only in areas of lining mucosa and not in future keratinizing regions. During this period the basement membrane becomes more clearly defined; hemi-desmosomes and basal lamina anchoring fibrils appear and in areas destined to become masticatory mucosa, epithelial rete ridges develop.

Nothing is known of the stage at which clear cells enter oral epithelium, but there is no reason to suppose that it differs from the epidermis into which the melanocytes appear to migrate from the 12th week onwards. Langerhans cells have been detected in epidermis from the same time and Merkel cells a little later, at the 16th week.

The development of the major salivary glands begins at about the 6th week from epithelial buds which invade the primitive mesenchyme. The minor salivary gland primordia are not apparent until the 8th week and grow as solid branching cords of epithelium, which later develop a lumen and thus form ducts. The secretory portion will later form around the ends of the finer ducts.

8:2 The control of mucosal development: epithelial-mesenchymal interaction

During embryological development cells are derived by mitotic division from the fertilized ovum. It is therefore reasonable to suggest that all cells initially possess the same genetic instructions but that during differentiation to form cells with different structures and functions, there is blocking of genetic material so that only information concerned with a particular pathway of differentiation is available to the cell. Blocking may well be a gradual process which proceeds until perhaps only one pathway of differentiation is left open. At this stage the cell may be said to be *determined*, determination simply representing the final step in a sequence of restrictive changes.

The actual process of differentiation is thought to be brought about by an *inductive mechanism* and there are many experiments, mostly based on tissues grown in organ culture, which suggest that the mesenchyme exerts a dominant controlling, or inductive, influence on epithelial differentiation. If the dermal component of embryonic skin is separated from the ectoderm, the ectoderm not only fails to differentiate but eventually dies. If recombined with its mesenchyme, then normal differentiation follows.

As all lining epithelia are continuously renewing cell populations the question arises as to whether this control continues to be exercised in subsequent generations of cells and eventually in adult tissues. Experimental evidence based upon the recombination and transplantation of dermal and epidermal components from various sites suggests that the dermis does appear to control the kind of epidermis growing at the graft site. This fact is of great importance to surgical procedures in man. For example, if skin is grafted into the mouth to replace an area of excised mucosa, it retains all the characteristics of the donor site, including hairs, because the dermis invariably forms part of the thickness of the graft. Likewise, in periodontal surgical procedures where flaps of oral mucosa are repositioned about the necks of teeth, the donor site determines the character of the newly positioned tissue; non-keratinized alveolar mucosa advanced to the gingiva will not take on the characteristics of the keratinized gingival mucosa in spite of altered functional demands at this site.

However, not all experiments have provided such clear cut evidence. For example, when epithelia from hamster tongue, palate and cheek pouch were combined with footpad dermis the epithelial specificity was retained. Trunk dermis, on the other hand, was able to induce tongue epithelium to form epidermis. These, and other experiments suggest that there may be a degree of *modulation* in the determination of epithelial character by the mesoderm.

Because signs of differentiation are more obvious in the epithelium than in the connective tissue, the latter is usually assumed to exercise the dominant influence. We cannot, however, discard the possibility that the epithelium might influence the mesenchyme, and evidence to this effect comes from organ culture experiments with developing tooth germs. At certain stages during early embryological development, the ectoderm appears to be dominant because, when ectoderm from the mouse molar region is recombined with incisor region mesenchyme, the morphology of the tooth which subsequently develops is characteristic of the ectodermal site. Later on, however, the mesenchyme again appears to determine tooth type.

The nature of the factors responsible for induction has been studied. Direct contact between the tissues is not essential for interaction to occur, as shown by the interpolation of microscopic membrane filters between tissue components in cultures of salivary glands, skin and teeth. Indeed the presence of living mesenchymal cells is not essential provided an extract of connective tissue is present and the epithelium has a suitable substratum on which to grow. It is clear that 'messenger molecules' must be involved and may be active over a considerable distance. These substances are both heat and trypsin labile and macromolecules such as RNA and proteoglycans have been suggested for this role.

8:3 Age changes in oral mucosa

All tissues undergo a series of gradual, inexorable and cumulative changes with age. These are perhaps best recognized in skin as the thinning and wrinkling of body skin, increased scaliness, the development of brown pigmented patches (lentigo) and spidery vascular naevi and, on the scalp, as greying of hair and baldness. Similar changes occur in oral mucosa which in the aged is comparatively thin, smooth and dry. Symptoms such as dryness, burning or itching, irregular roughness and abnormal taste are common, particularly in post-menopausal women. As tissues in the aged recover less readily from injury, and particularly as most old people are edentulous, degenerative changes in the oral mucosa are of great practical importance.

Age changes may well be programmed by the genetic material of the cells in much the same way as the fertilized ovum carries a programme for the development of the whole organism. Indeed programmed cell death plays an important part in embryonic development, for example that which occurs in the ectodermal lining of the palatal shelves prior to fusion of their mesenchymal components. Furthermore there is experimental evidence from tissue culture studies that the number of divisions of which a population of fibroblasts is capable is pre-determined by the cells themselves; the older the donor the fewer the divisions that are possible and for cells derived from various animals, the number of divisions is proportional to the normal life span of the species.

In studying oral mucosa it is difficult to determine to what extent the age changes seen are the inevitable result of this kind of programmed senescence, and to what extent they are secondary to local wear and tear and to systemic factors such as changes in blood supply, nutrition and hormonal activity.

Age changes in oral mucosa and skin are naturally similar, and most of the available evidence is derived from studies on skin. Some of the evidence is contra-dictory, arising from failure adequately to account for regional variations and for intercurrent disease or, for example, from the wearing of dentures, smoking and other environmental influences; nevertheless the general sequence of events is clear. There is generalized atrophy of mucosa and skin with age; the epithelium becomes thinner overall, individual layers varying in thickness and regularity, and there is disparity in size and shape of individual cells and of their nuclei. There is a reduc-tion or simplification of the epithelial rete ridges so that the epithelium-connective tissue junction becomes flatter, and the basement membrane becomes thinner and irregular.

Clinical observation and histology suggest that this atrophic epithelium shows increasing keratinization with age. This is most obvious on normally non-keratinized lining mucosa, and on the vermilion border of the lip, and is characteristically irregular in distri-bution leading to the formation of white plaques and complaints of roughness. As malignancy in oral mucosa is sometimes preceded by keratosis and as oral cancer, like most forms of malignancy, is more common in the elderly, such areas should be observed closely and if suspicion is aroused, biopsied for histopathological examination.

The specialized mucosa of the dorsum of the tongue is particularly prone to atrophy, with marked loss of fili-form papillae, and this is often predisposed to by nutri-tional deficiency, particularly of iron and of B-group vitamins, which may be common in undernourished elderly persons, and by pernicious anaemia.

Many of the changes referred to above, most notably atrophy and keratosis, are found in post-menopausal women and mirror changes in genital mucosae. They

107

may be reversed to some extent by administration of oestrogen.

The structural changes associated with age may be a reflection of changes in epithelial cell dynamics, but the evidence is conflicting. It has been suggested that mitotic activity is increased in aged oral mucosa but mitotic counts in human tissue, where mitotic arrest techniques cannot be used, are not very accurate. Furthermore, if mitotic counts are expressed as a proportion of the total cells present in a given region of tissue, the results will be distorted by the atrophic character of the epithelium. More recent work, employing thymidine-labelling techniques and studies of the phases of the cell cycle indicate that the duration of mitosis is increased, and there is an overall slowing of tissue turnover; this is what would be expected from the general reduction in metabolic activity of all tissues with age. There may be an increase in the number of recognizable clear cells within epithelium with age, but many of these may be inflammatory cells, and it is known that the average number of melanocytes per unit area of skin surface actually decreases throughout life, by approximately 11% per decade.

The cellularity of the lamina propria of the oral mucosa is substantially decreased in old age. All cell types appear to be involved, the fibroblasts in particular becoming shrunken with condensed, elongate nuclei and scanty cytoplasm. This is associated with a decrease in the amount of ground substance and with degeneration, fragmentation and hyalinization of collagen—a condition sometimes called hyaline degeneration. A progressive increase in inter- and intra-molecular cross links can be demonstrated in aged collagen, with consequent alteration in its physical properties.

In contrast, elastic fibres are said to increase with age, particularly in exposed areas of skin where the condition is called senile, or solar, elastosis. This is in conflict with the observed decreased elasticity of aged skin and the paradox can be explained by the fact that, as part of its own age change, collagen tends to stain with the standard stains for elastin. This altered collagen, termed collastin, does not have the chemical or physical properties of elastin, and electron microscopy reveals that true elastic fibres become split and fragmented with advancing age.

Changes in the vasculature of the oral mucosa are common in the elderly. Some degree of arteriosclerosis is often seen and a striking feature may be nodular, varicose enlargement of the superficial veins on the under surface of the tongue, known as caviar tongue. Similar, but smaller, vascular nodules as well as redder capillary naevi, tend to occur also in the mucosa of the lips and cheeks, like the spidery naevi that occur on the skin, the conjunctiva and nail bed in advanced age.

The number of sebaceous glands in the lips and cheeks may increase quite markedly in old age, producing large Fordyce's spots. In contrast, there is usually marked atrophy of the minor salivary glands, which contain few functional acini and increased fibrous tissue and fat. In all salivary tissue there is a progressive increase in the number of oncocytes—distinctive cells with a large amount of eosinophilic granular cytoplasm. Diffuse infiltrations of lymphocytes are common in the glands of up to 70% of persons over 45 years of age, although in the absence of salivary gland disease, the prevalence does not increase further with advancing age. Larger deposits of fat may appear in association with the minor salivary glands of the soft palate and, in aged people, may extend as confluent yellow patches to the anterior pillar of the fauces and the retromolar areas.

The density of nerve endings decreases with advancing age in both skin and oral mucosa, particularly in gingiva and tongue, and taste buds are much reduced. The whole range of sensory nerves, including those of proprioceptive function is likely to be involved, and this is consistent with the observation that there is loss of power to perceive and discriminate between tastes in the elderly, and that adaptation to denture wearing is much more difficult than in younger individuals.

Further reading

KOLLAR E.J. (1972) Histogenetic aspects of dermal-epidermal interactions. In *Developmental Aspects of Oral Biology* (edited by Slavkin, H.C. and Bavetta, L.A.) 126–150. Academic Press, New York.

MILES A.E.W. (1972) 'Sans Teeth': changes in the oral tissues with advancing age. *Proc. Roy Soc. Med.* **69**, 801–806.

VAN WYK C.W. (1970 The development of keratin in the human mouth. *J. dent. Ass. S. Africa* **25**, 348–352.

SUPPLEMENTARY READING

A good account of the histology of human oral mucosa, including regional variations, is to be found in:

SICHER H. & BHASKAR S.N. (1972) *Orban's Oral Histology and Embryology.* 7th Edition. C.V. Mosby Company, St. Louis.

Many of the topics in this volume are dealt with in more detail in:

MELCHER A.H. & BOWEN W.H. (Eds.) (1969) *Biology of the Periodontium.* Academic Press, London.
SQUIER C.A. & MEYER J. (Eds.) (1971) *Current Concepts of the Histology of Oral Mucosa.* Charles C. Thomas, Springfield, Illinois.

Concise authoritative accounts of various aspects of the oral mucosa are included in:

COHEN B. & KRAMER I.R.H. (Eds.) (1976) *Scientific Foundations of Dentristry.* Wm. Heinemann Medical Books, London.

A more comprehensive treatment of physiology and immunology as well as of disease processes affecting the oral mucosa are contained in:

DOLBY A.E. (Ed.) (1975) *Oral Mucosa in Health and Disease.* Blackwell Scientific Publications, Oxford.

111

Two books on skin which contain much that is relevant to considerations of development and morphology of the oral mucosa are:

BREATHNACH A.S. (1971) *An Atlas of Ultrastructure of Human Skin; development, differentiation and post-natal features.* J. & A. Churchill, London.
MONTAGNA W. & PARAKKAL P.F. (1974) *The Structure and Function of Skin.* 3rd Edition. Academic Press, New York.

APPENDIX 1
TECHNIQUES FOR PREPARING
TISSUES FOR MICROSCOPICAL
EXAMINATION

1:1 Histological techniques

Methods to prepare tissues for histological examination have been developed continuously for over 150 years and there are numerous texts that deal with this topic very fully. What follows is an extremely brief account of the main steps involved in routine histological preparations.

In order to examine tissue with the light microscope it is usually necessary to prepare slices or sections thin enough (usually 5–7 µm) to permit adequate transmission of light through the specimen, and then to differentially stain the constituents of the tissue so as to introduce contrast between the various cellular and tissue elements. This involves a sequence of events in which the fresh material is first *fixed* chemically (usually with a formaldehyde solution) to prevent autolysis and to render many of the tissue components insoluble. The next stage involves infiltration with a supporting medium which permeates the cells and intercellular regions so as to permit *sectioning* on a microtome. As the most commonly used embedding medium, paraffin wax, is not water soluble the specimens must be dehydrated in increasing concentrations of alcohol before being infiltrated with the molten wax. There are occasions when thinner sections are required or when particularly tough or heterogeneous tissue has to be embedded, in which case harder waxes, celloidin or even epoxy resins may be used.

Table 6. Common histological and histochemical stains.

	Stain	To demonstrate	Appearance
Histological stains	*Van Gieson*	Collagen	Red
	Weigert's orcein (resorcin fuchsin)	Elastin	Purple-black
	Metal Impregnation (Au, Ag, Os) e.g. Gomori silver	Reticulin	Brown-black
	Masson, argentaffin reaction	Melanin	Black
	Bielschowsky method	Nerves	Brown-black
	Papanicolaou	Types of keratinization	Keratinized epithelium: keratin, red-orange; Malpighian cells, green; non-keratinized epithelium: green
	Methyl green-pyronin	Plasma cells and other cells with high content of cytoplasmic RNA	Bright pink cytoplasm, blue-green nucleus

Table 6. Continued.

Stain	To demonstrate	Appearance
Histochemical stains		
Periodic acid-Schiff (paS)	Carbohydrates such as glycogen; glycoproteins including basement membrane	Bright pink
Alcian blue	Proteoglycans, some glycoproteins	Turquoise-blue
Metachromatic dyes e.g. toluidine blue crystal violet	Proteoglycans e.g. ground substance, mast cell granules, amyloid	Toluidine blue–purple metachromasia Crystal violet–red metachromasia
Feulgen reaction	D.N.A.	Purple
Enzyme methods		
Hydrolases e.g. acid phosphatase alkaline phosphatase	Lysosomes in macrophages etc. Plasma membranes particularly around capillaries, specific granules of polymorphonuclear leucocytes	Reaction product will depend on method used: metal precipitation methods yield brown-black end products, azo dye methods produce brightly coloured end products
A.T.Pase	Plasma membranes	
Oxido-reductases e.g. succinic dehydrogenase lactic dehydrogenase cytochrome oxidase	Respiratory pathways particularly in epithelium	
dihydroxyphenylalanine (dopa) oxidase	Melanin synthesis	

Mineralized tissue, such as tooth or bone, is difficult to cut on a normal microtome and so must usually be demineralized before embedding. This is carried out by using dilute acids or a chelating agent such as ethylene diamine tetra-acetic acid (EDTA).

Sections of embedded tissue are mounted on glass microscope slides and the embedding medium removed with a solvent such as xylene. They can then be rehydrated so as to permit *staining* with any of a variety of aqueous dyes before being again dehydrated and *mounted* in a transparent liquid medium such as Canada balsam or polystyrene resin such as DPX, which then form a permanent preparation.

The most common staining routine is to use haematoxylin and eosin. Haematoxylin is a *basophilic* stain, having an affinity for acid structures such as nucleic acids and certain mucosubstances. Eosin is *acidophilic* and stains basic groups, such as those of the proteins, collagen, keratin and haemoglobin. Where more information about particular cell or tissue constituents is required numerous other staining methods may be used, and some of these are listed in Table 6.

1:1:1 HISTOCHEMISTRY

Most histological staining methods are based on a chemical or physical interaction between dye and tissue, but as the basis of these methods is rarely understood, they do not convey much information about the chemical nature of biological structure. Histochemistry is concerned with the microscopic localization and identification of compounds within cells or tissues without loss of their structural integrity. A variety of substances can be demonstrated in this way, such as lipids, nucleic acids, proteins and carbohydrates including mucosubstances. It represents a meeting point between biochemistry and histology, for although histochemistry lacks the full quantitative and dynamic advantages of the former, it contributes a functional aspect to the static nature of histology.

Material must be prepared for histochemistry so as to ensure the least damage to the tissue or to the compound being investigated. Although chemical fixation and routine histological processing may be used these procedures tend to destroy many biological substances, such

116

as enzymes, and it is commonplace initially to freeze the tissue and prepare sections using a freezing microtome or *cryostat*. The sections can then be reacted under appropriate conditions to obtain a stable, coloured end-product that is sharply localized. The most widely used methods are for demonstrating enzymes involved in hydrolytic or oxidation/reduction reactions (see Table 6).

1:1:2 MICROCHEMISTRY

This is more akin to biochemistry than are most histo-chemical methods. Fragments of freeze-dried tissue are weighed and incubated with substrate and the soluble reaction products estimated quantitatively by standard spectrophotometric methods.

1:2 Electron microscope techniques

The electron microscope, by using electrons which have a far shorter wavelength than visible light, provides much higher resolution than is attainable in the light microscope. The methods for preparing sections for examination in the *transmission electron microscope* (TEM) are not unlike those of histology, but have been modified to cope with the rather stringent requirements of the instrument. Normal electron microscopes do not produce an electron beam with sufficient energy to pene-trate sections much thicker than 100 nm (0·1 μm) and must operate under high vacuum conditions. Moreover at the greater magnifications achieved within the elec-tron microscope fixation by normal histological methods is not adequate.

The first requirement for adequate fixation and em-bedding for electron microscopy is that specimens must be very much smaller than those used for histology, and preferably no larger than 1 mm cubes. Fixatives that are routinely used are buffered formaldehyde-glutaraldehyde mixtures or solutions of osmium tetroxide. This latter agent not only fixes tissue but also selectively introduces electron dense atoms of osmium into the specimen, which serve to increase contrast. After dehydration, the specimens are usually embedded in an epoxy resin which on polymerization produces an extremely tough and hard block. These blocks are sectioned, using diamond or glass knives, on an *ultramicrotome*, a specially designed instrument capable of producing sections, under optimum conditions, that may be as thin as 40 nm.

Finally the sections are collected on to small nickel or copper grids when they may be 'stained' by immersing in solutions of lead or uranium salts. These metals, like osmium, are selectively taken up by the tissues, and impart contrast by scattering the electron beam.

Scanning electron microscopy (SEM) utilizes the primary electrons scattered, and the secondary electrons emitted, from the surface of a solid object to provide a detailed picture of that surface. In this case sectioning is clearly not necessary, but in order to resist distortion under the high vacuum of the microscope, specimens must first be fixed and dehydrated. Finally the surface has to be coated with a conducting layer to prevent charging of the specimen by the bombarding electrons. This can be carried out by evaporating onto the specimen an extremely thin film of carbon followed by gold or platinum.

Further reading

BAKER J.R. (1969) *Cytological Technique* (4th edition) Science Paperbacks, Associated Book Publishers, London.

BOYDE A. & WOOD C. (1969) Preparation of animal tissues for surface scanning electron microscopy. *J. Microscopy* **90**, 221–249.

GERSON S. & MEYER J. (1970) Biochemical assay of heterogeneous soft tissues of the oral cavity. *Advances in Oral Biology* **4**, 289–312.

MERCER E.H. & BIRBECK M.S.C. (1966) *Electron microscopy: a handbook for biologists* (2nd edition) Blackwell Scientific Publications, Oxford.

APPENDIX 2
MUCOSUBSTANCES

2:1 Classification

A number of substances produced by the body consist of complex macromolecules containing both proteins and carbohydrates. Familiar examples are epithelial intercellular cement substance, the ground substance of connective tissue and the mucous secretions of the gastrointestinal tract. The chemical classification of these different substances has often been confused, different workers using different names to describe the same substance. In an attempt to clarify this situation, the general and chemically non-committal title of mucosubstance has been given to all these protein-carbohydrate complexes.

This term encompasses both *glycoproteins* (sometimes referred to as mucoproteins, sialomucins or sialomucopolysaccharides) and *proteoglycans* (mucopolysaccharides). The term glycosaminoglycans is sometimes used to refer to the carbohydrate moiety of proteoglycans.

Both glycoproteins and proteoglycans are thought to contain a single polypeptide chain which forms a backbone to which oligo—or polysaccharide chains are covalently attached. Whereas the glycoproteins, which are predominantly protein in character, often (but not invariably) have a relatively small carbohydrate component, proteoglycans contain a large proportion of carbohydrate and thus behave more like polysaccharides than proteins. In distinguishing between the two classes

Table 7. Characteristics of carbohydrate side chains of glycoproteins and proteoglycans.

			Glycoproteins	Proteoglycans
Length			2–15 sugar residues	150–several thousand sugar residues
Nature			Often branched	Always linear
Regularity/ homogeneity			There is no repeating sequence of sugar residues. Side chains need not be identical and molecules of the same glycoprotein may be heterogeneous	Contains a regular repeating sequence of 2 sugar residues, one of which is usually a hexosamine, the other a hexuronic acid
Characteristic sugar residues	Simple hexoses		D-galactose D-mannose D-glucose	D-galactose — —
	Simple pentoses		L-arabinose D-xylose	— —
	De-oxy sugars (when present always occupy terminal position in side chain)		L-fucose N-acetylneuraminic acid (sialic acid)	— —
	hexosamines		N-acetyl-D-glucosamine N-acetyl-D-galactosamine	N-acetyl-D-glucosamine N-acetyl-D-galactosamine
	hexosamine sulphates		— — —	N-acetyl-D-galactosamine 4-SO_4 N-acetyl-D-galactosamine 6-SO_4 N-acetyl-D-glucosamine 6-SO_4
	hexuronic acids		— —	D-glucuronic acid L-iduronic acid

of mucosubstances, it is the nature of the carbohydrate side chains that is important. Some of the more important characteristics of these carbohydrate components are shown in Table 7.

Some examples of commonly occurring mucosubstances and their synonyms are listed below.

Glycoproteins	Salivary mucins
	Blood group substances
	Collagen
	Interferon
	Ribonuclease B

Proteoglycans	Chondroitin	
	Chondroitin Sulphate A	(Chondroitin-4- sulphate)
	Chondroitin Sulphate B	(Dermatan sulphate)
	Chondroitin Sulphate C	(Chondroitin-6- sulphate)
	Keratan sulphate	(Keratosulphate)
	Heparan sulphate	(Heparatin sulphate)
	Hyaluronic acid	

While most mucosubstances will fit into the classification shown in Table 7 there are inevitably exceptions and it is possible for some mucosubstances to have side chains of both types.

2:2 Staining characteristics

Failing a complete biochemical analysis, the most common means of distinguishing between mucosubstances is by the application of histological staining methods. For the histopathologist this may be the only means of recognition.

Unless a glycoprotein contains a sialic acid residue (which if present is always situated at the free end of a carbohydrate side chain) it will be neutrally charged. On the other hand, proteoglycans all carry a net negative charge due to the presence of sulphate and/or carboxy-groups. These differences in charge account in part for the different histochemical staining reactions shown by the two groups of substances. Thus proteoglycans and also glycoproteins containing sialic acid will stain non-specifically with cationic dyes such as toluidine blue, alcian blue or ruthenium red. However, because proteoglycans contain a regular repeating anionic structure, they alone will stain *metachromatically* with dyes such as toluidine blue or crystal violet. That is to say, during the binding of these stains a change occurs in their absorption spectrum so that they appear a different colour from the original dye.

On the other hand, glycoproteins, including those containing sialic acid residues, can be stained by the periodic acid-Schiff (paS) technique. This method depends upon oxidation of adjacent glycol groups with periodic acid followed by reaction of the dialdehydes so formed with Schiff's base. Under controlled conditions this staining procedure is relatively specific for glycoproteins, and proteoglycans are said not to stain by this method.

More specific identification of mucosubstances can be made by the use of stains specific for sulphate esters or uronic acids and by digestion of sections with the appropriate enzymes.

Further reading

BARRETT A.J. (1971) The biochemistry and function of mucosub-stances. *Histochem. J.* 3, 213–221.

INDEX

124

125